USING STRATEGIC AND TACTICAL PLANNING TO MAKE YOUR VETERINARY PRACTICE MORE PROFITABLE

A PRIMER

Brian M. Hayden

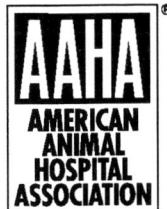

AAHA®
AMERICAN
ANIMAL
HOSPITAL
ASSOCIATION

Many thanks to the AAHA Press Editorial Advisory Board:
Dr. Laurel Collins, ABVP
Dr. Richard Goebel
Dr. Charles Hickey
Dr. Clayton McKinnon
Dr. Richard Nelson, ABVP
Dr. Hal Taylor

AAHA Press
12575 W. Bayaud Avenue
Lakewood, Colorado 80228

ISBN: 1-58326-019-6

This book is dedicated to my first grandson,
Conner, who was born on June 8, 1999.
It just goes to show that even without planning,
wonderful things can still happen.

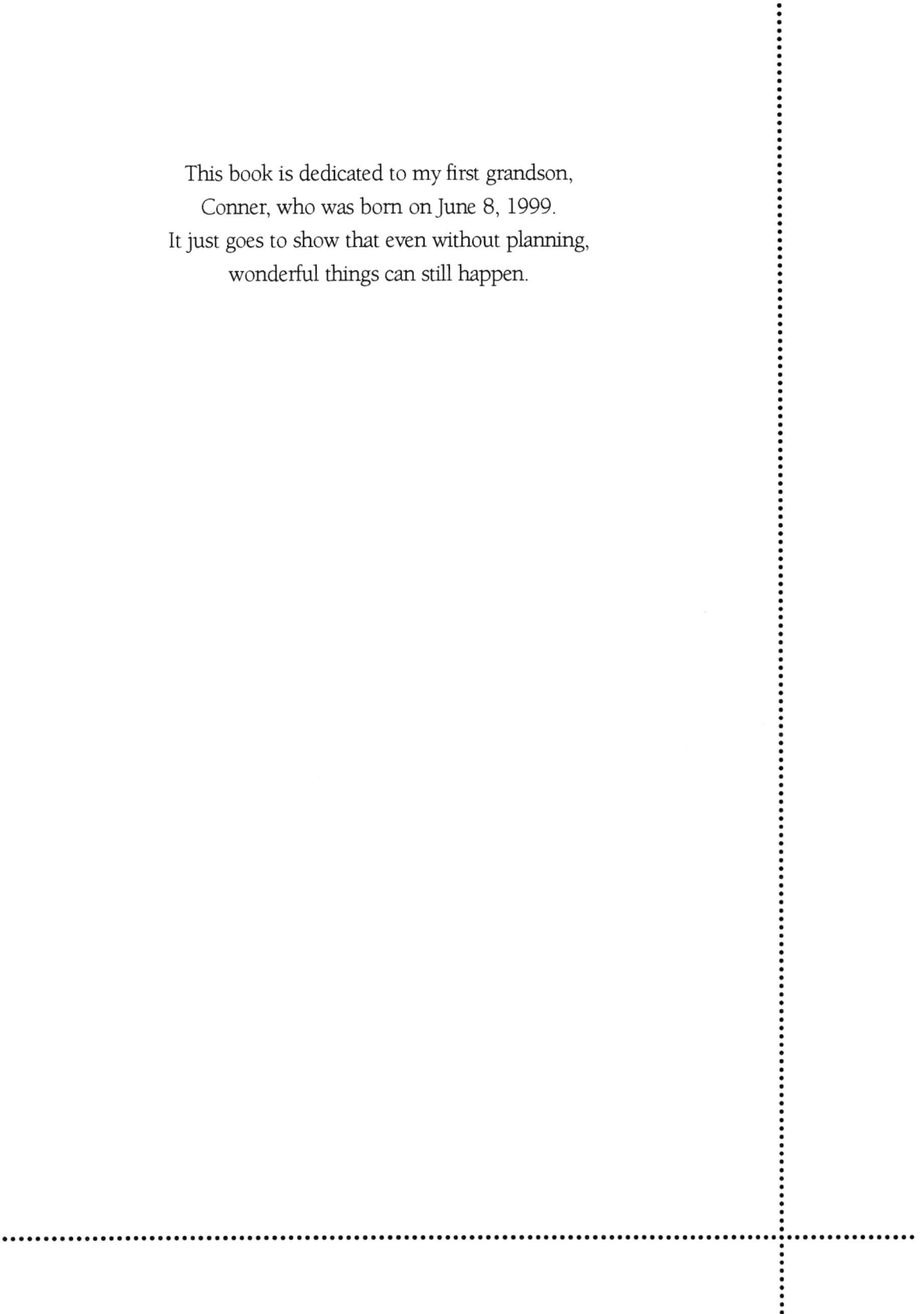

CONTENTS

FIGURES

PREFACE

This was never supposed to be a book. I was simply going to provide guidelines for some folks I met at a national meeting. I recognized that over time, many receptionists, technicians, and veterinarians found themselves in key management roles—roles they accepted but were not really trained to do. My intention was to help them understand the process of planning and show them how it could help them.

So I started writing down some thoughts on planning. The thoughts flowed like water. I was a writing fool! Within two days I had created a 24-page booklet. It was a proud moment, so I shared my work with a couple of coworkers. As I began getting feedback, it became apparent that I had stumbled on an idea for a book. Oh yes, there are plenty of books about planning, but none that I've found that speak to an audience of veterinary managers and veterinarians who have had no formal management training.

So here it is—the book on understanding strategic and tactical planning written for those of you who are managing veterinary hospitals and clinics every day, those of you who are striving to be more profitable, working diligently to accomplish the myriad of things that need to be done. I'm proud to give you a tool that will make your life a bit less confusing and a whole lot more productive.

Brian Hayden

ACKNOWLEDGMENTS

I would like to thank a number of people without whose help this book would not have come to fruition. Thank you to Susan Milner and Shannon Miller, who volunteered to read the first notes I wrote while developing this project. Your feedback was instrumental in helping me clarify my ideas.

A very sincere thank you to Anne Serrano, the acquisitions editor, whose words of encouragement kept me going and whose assistance in organizing my book proved invaluable.

To my father, Paul Hayden, thank you for all the times you told me I could do whatever I set my mind to. Guess you were right! Lastly, a very special thanks to my family: my son, Joseph, my daughter, Angela, and my wife of 25 years, Denise. I've spent many years away from home in search of bigger and better jobs. You gave me the support and patience I needed to follow my career. Any success I achieve is a direct result of your encouragement, support, and love.

Using Strategic and Tactical Planning to Make Your Veterinary Practice More Profitable

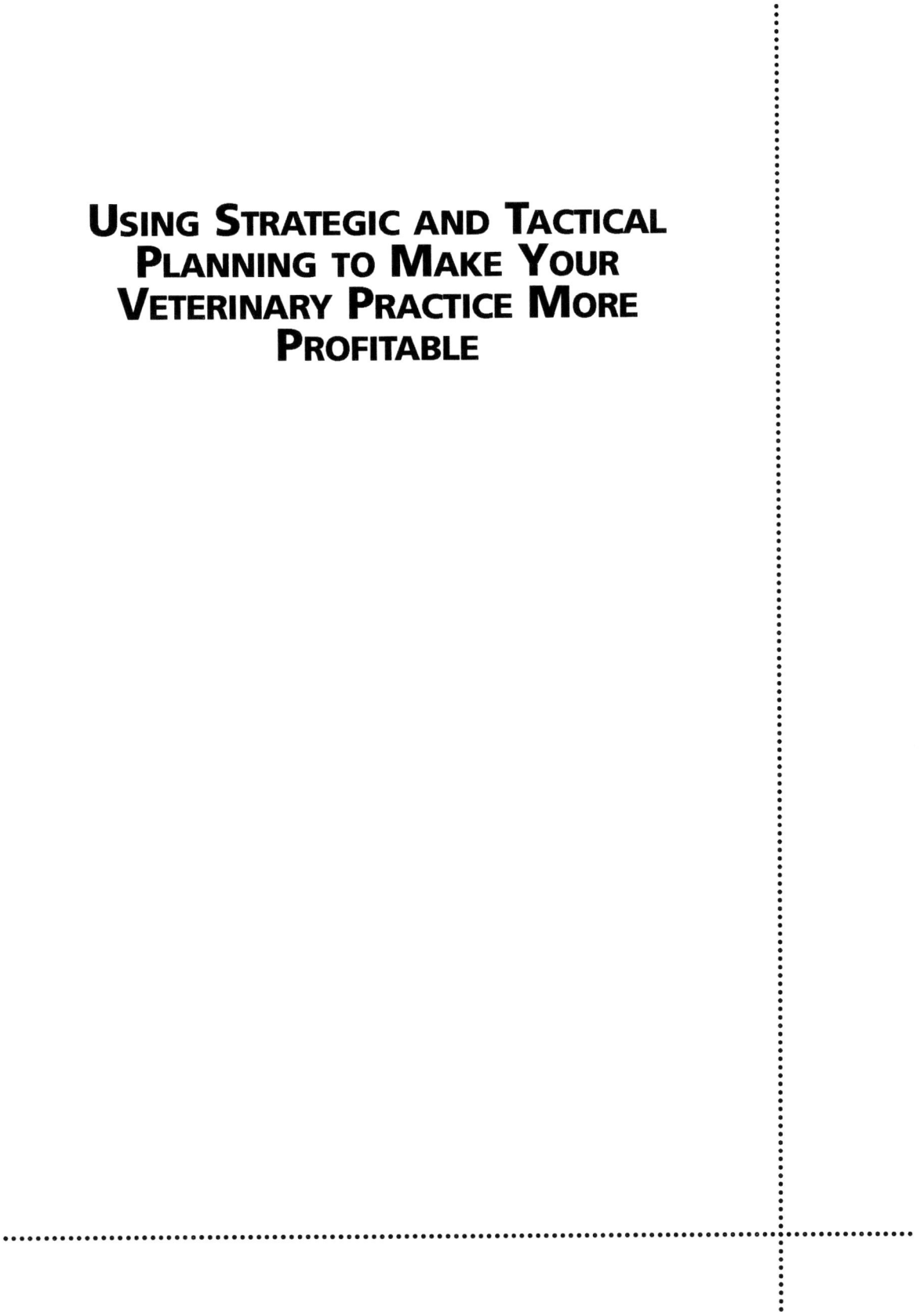

CHAPTER 1

INTRODUCTION

"Failing to plan is a plan for failure."

Having come from a military background (retired Air Force), I was used to planning; it was just something we did—an integral part of my everyday schedule. As I made the transition into the commercial veterinary environment, the planning process came right along. I hardly thought about it... that is until a fateful day last January. As I walked into the hospital, I was immediately set upon by a receptionist who wanted to know what she was supposed to tell clients about our February dental special. Apparently, some of our more loyal clients knew they could get good deals on dental exams for their pets in February and had already begun calling.

To be honest I had forgotten! So like the good manager I tell people I am, I did what needed to be done. I quickly called a meeting of my management group. After the last of my managers found their seats, I began asking questions: "What do you mean the dental special is coming up in two days?" "What's going to be in it?" "How will it work?" "Who's going to do the flyers?" "The sign?" "How will we track its success?"

Nobody had the answers. So I shifted into crisis management mode and after a day of aggravation, we were ready. As I sat at my kitchen table that night reflecting over the day's events, it occurred to me that I wouldn't have been in such a tight situation if only I'd planned a little better. Oh sure, we had mentioned the special once—briefly—in the strategic business plan listed in obscurity under Marketing Calendar. But we had never figured out precisely what we were going to do, who was going to do it, how much it would cost us, and when everything needed to be done. In other words, we hadn't prepared a tactical plan. We had failed to complete the total business plan. Far too often we neglect the essential step of tactical planning—the part that answers the questions: Who, Where, When, How, and How Much—you know, the step that helps us succeed!

Making tactical plans is critical for managers at all veterinary facilities, regardless of size. I've run hospitals from the one-man, $15,000-a-month type to the multimillion-dollar, 24-hour operation and everything in between. I assure you, tactical planning is important to all. For years, managers at many different levels have ignored the tactical planning process. If they did undertake some type of tactical plan, they didn't realize it. It was an accident. Did you ever notice that middle and upper managers usually have gray hair? I've noticed, and I can't help but think that if those managers used tactical planning in a deliberate, purposeful manner, their hair might still be the original color.

In the veterinary industry, we are in double trouble. First, doctors often manage our clinics and hospitals. Now that's not to say there aren't doctors who are good managers. There are! Some of the best managers I know are doctors. However, the managing doctor who also wants to practice medicine is faced with a problem. There just isn't enough time to properly perform both jobs. Often the doctor gets involved in patient care, and the planning process goes out the window. Alternatively, the doctor gets into patient care, then spends an additional four to eight hours a day to keep up with the management functions of the job. What kind of life is that? Twelve hours a day or more! I see burnout in their futures. Second, professional hospital managers, although often very talented, aren't usually formally trained in management. That's not to say they don't do a good job. Most do! But their lack of formal management training may be the cause of some stress and loss of productivity. They may not have the tools to get everything done efficiently.

I know that's true because I've been guilty of the same errors. Sometimes I was caught up in doing so many things that I neglected doing the one thing that would have helped me the most—making a tactical plan! That's part of the impetus behind this book. I want to give you a tool that can make your life easier and make you much more productive. If you recognize the importance of tactical plans, learn how to use them, and use them to their fullest extent, you will have success in your practice, you will be more productive, and your blood pressure will probably go down. All of which are good reasons to implement tactical plans in your practice! Imagine, if you will, what your life at work would be like without so many surprises—you'd come to work knowing what's going to happen and having all those projects and chores that need to be done organized, prioritized, delegated, and set up in such a way that you can easily track your progress. A comforting thought, isn't it? We all think that we can remember to do all that needs to be done. *The reality is we don't.* We get good ideas and say to ourselves, "This idea can really make some money." The reality is we get pulled in other directions to put out a fire or to handle another crisis, and we don't follow through on our idea. How often have you intended to do something but never gotten around to it? If you're like most of us, you probably answered that question, "Too often."

Understanding tactical planning and how to implement tactical plans will help you take some of the chaos out of your life. Have you ever felt the practice was running you? Aren't you supposed to be running the practice? Tactical plans will help you regain control, will help you to remember to get projects done, and will provide you with a method of tracking your progress. When projects get done, productivity increases. When you reduce the time you spend putting out fires, your productivity goes up. When productivity goes up, your profits will surely follow. What a glorious day it will be when you can combine doing a job you love with making money!

Owning the practice, or being charged with the responsibility for running a practice, carries a responsibility most don't recognize—the employees, who share our love and compassion for animals and rejoice in the opportunity to care for them. Most of them are not in the profession for the money, so it becomes incumbent upon us to make their careers as rewarding as possible. To give your employees a rewarding career you must develop a thriving business, become profitable, and generate enough money to pay them well. The key to doing that is to become proficient in planning. In this book, I'll explain tactical planning and give you many examples and exercises to reinforce the lessons. To help ensure your success, I'll also provide detailed explanations of how to implement the plans. It's one thing to read about a technique and quite another to make it happen. Before we discuss tactical planning, however, we need to discuss strategic planning. For it is within the strategic plans that the tactical plans are born. There are dozens of books that discuss strategic plans, and I do not intend to rehash the subject. Once you understand strategic planning, you'll be able to make the transition to the tactical plans. Then you will begin to understand the power of planning and the significant impact proper planning can have on your ability to practice profitably.

CHAPTER 2

STRATEGIC PLANNING

"If you want to finish that elephant on your plate, you gotta do it one bite at a time."

As I said before, much of my experience as an administrator was gained in the military. Although the military isn't a commercial enterprise, its job is broad in scope. The need for strategic planning in any multifaceted environment increases almost exponentially with increased tasks. As practices and business systems become more complex, planning becomes a necessity.

Strategic Plans: A Vision Quest

Creating a strategic plan is the crucial first step in the planning process. Strategic plans lay the foundation for everything you want your hospital to achieve. If you think it sounds like goal-setting, you are right. Writing a strategic plan is a vision quest. Not only does it help you set goals and clarify your vision for the practice, it can also help you define the level of achievement to which you aspire. As you begin to dig into strategic planning, you'll discover it also becomes an important tool for assessing where you are, which is essential because you can't know how to get where you want to be unless you know where you are now.

You may already begin to see that strategic plans, if done correctly, are powerful. That's why so many books are written about them. Our economy is good—even great—now. But how long will it last? Using strategic planning in a good economy will propel your practice above those practices without strategic plans. Using strategic planning in a weak economy may be the difference between success and a slip into mediocrity. But like most things, the art of proper planning requires knowledge and takes practice. We'll begin by examining and understanding strategic plans.

The Importance of Self-Evaluation

To figure out where you are today, you need to do a self-evaluation. I believe that an honest, detailed self-evaluation is the most important part of the strategic plan. As the old saying goes, "You can't fix it if you don't know it's broke." You'll soon see, that knowing in great detail how everything in your practice is working will go further toward helping you achieve your goals than just about anything else I know. Of course, having baseline data on your practice will also help you to set your goals. It's easy to say you want an average transaction of $100. But if your current transaction average is sitting at $55, it might not be realistic to set your goal at $100. You can see that knowing where you are now will help you set realistic, attainable goals; but a self-evaluation does so much more than that. It will become the foundation for writing your plan.

Using the format that I outline will cast a whole new light on your practice. It may not always be a pleasing light, but it will give you a good feeling because you'll have a handle on how things really are in your business. It will lay out what needs to be fixed and how to fix it. That's when the evaluation becomes powerful. That's when you'll begin to feel you have control over your practice—your business. And that is what this book is all about—regaining control of your practice and making it work as efficiently and effectively as possible. I'll provide you with plenty of examples as well as a number of exercises that will reinforce the concepts. In addition, several forms, inspection checklists, and appendixes are included to help you. I do know how difficult the process can be because I am a practicing administrator of animal hospitals. I also know what you need, and I'm pretty sure I know how to get that information to you. Let's dig into the strategic plan and try to make some sense out of it.

Defining *Strategic Plan*

Far too often people use words without really knowing what they mean. So let's stop for a moment to understand what we're talking about. Sometimes we fall into a trap. Instead of looking at the component words, we see the whole unit (*strategic plan*, in this case) and derive a meaning from it. That approach would be a big mistake here. To understand what strategic plan means, you need to break it down. Let's start by looking at *strategic plan* as two distinct words.

Defining *Plan*

Since I rarely do things in the traditional way, let's start by looking at the second word first. The dictionary gives us about twenty or so meanings of *plan*. I've selected the ones I consider the top four.

- A method for achieving an end
- A detailed formulation of a program of action
- Goal, aim
- An orderly arrangement of parts of an overall design or objective

Those meanings are probably the ones most of you already knew. It's also probably no surprise to you that there are lots of different types of plans. We use adjectives to describe the type of plan we're talking about: vacation plans, retirement plans, travel plans, strategic plans. Now all we have to do is figure out what *strategic* means. For that, we go back to the dictionary.

Defining *Strategic*

Again, there are a variety of definitions of *strategic*. This is the one I like: "necessary to or important in the initiation, conduct or completion of a plan." But what does it mean in reality? You have a business that is called your practice. You have certain expectations for your practice—your goals. But there are so many things to do to accomplish your goals that you can't keep them all in your head. So you begin to write them down. Then you figure out what you have to do to accomplish your goals. You write that down, too. Finally, you shift into overdrive and make a timetable to accomplish the things that need to be done. You've just written a strategic plan! You wrote down the steps necessary to reach your goals. You developed a timetable that was important to the initiation of your plan. You wrote down the steps needed to complete your plan. Strategic plans lay out your goals, identify the actions required to meet your goals, and put all of it in a timetable for you to follow. That's it! Who would have thought a phrase as imposing as *strategic plans* could be so simple. Now all we need to do is identify some basic parts of the strategic business plan and we're on the road.

Components of the Strategic Plan

Strategic plans have three primary parts: self-evaluation, action lists, and budgets. I'm not going to discuss budgets in this book, although it is important to recognize that budgets are an integral part of the strategic planning process and that they complete the picture we'll be drawing of a practice. To get more information on budgeting, you can refer to many fine books written on the subject. You can also check with a certified public accountant or a veterinary practice consultant. For our purposes, we'll concentrate on the self-evaluation and on the action lists. We'll look at each one individually and then see how they relate and work with each other.

Self-Evaluation: Strengths, Weaknesses, and Assessment

The self-evaluation is the foundation of any good strategic plan. In my interpretation of the self-evaluation we have three key parts: strengths, weaknesses, and assessment. First, you identify what's right and what's wrong—your strengths and weaknesses. Next, you look at that information and provide an assessment. Finally, you compile action lists. But I don't want to get ahead of myself, so I'll put that on the back burner for now. Let's break down the self-evaluation process into its parts and discuss each one.

Before we begin our discussion of a self-evaluation and, more concisely, an assessment, I must make mention of the issue of honesty. An evaluation has no value if you're not totally honest. I'm not talking about "mostly" or "usually" or "sometimes." I'm talking about blunt, brutal honesty. If you are not prepared to be totally honest with your-self about how your practice is performing, you are wasting your time. It's only through the frank appraisal of your operating systems that the whole process will be effective. You must be sincere in your quest for the truth. Then, and only then, can the appraisal process be telling. The caveat about being honest applies even if you are not an owner of a practice but are part of the corporate structure. If you write a strategic plan, you should be giving the owner or corporate heads a clear picture of what's going on in the business. Beware of the consequences of being dishonest. Do not be tempted to lie. I once knew a manager who gave himself glowing comments in the evaluation process. Our corporate headquarters was in another state, so I guess he didn't think that individuals at headquarters would ever check the veracity of his report—he was wrong. When they started reviewing his report with him, it became clear that things weren't as good as he had depicted. I'm not sure but I think he's a waiter now!

"You can fool a fool some of the time, but if you try to fool your boss, you'll probably get fired."

Remember I said self-evaluation consisted of three parts: strengths, weaknesses, and assessment. The assessment is a narrative summary of the strengths and weaknesses of one part of the self-evaluation checklist. It is the honest appraisal of each function within the practice. Appendix A (p. 89) shows a self-evaluation checklist that breaks down the components of a typical hospital into bite-sized pieces. As you go through the checklist evaluating your practice, you'll be making notes about the things you are doing right and the things that require improvement. You will also note some of the areas in which you really excel—your strengths. The areas that require improvement are your weaknesses. In assessing the situation, pretend you are explaining your findings to an individual sitting across a table from you. If you write the assessment as you would speak to that person, you will provide a very clear picture. Keep in mind, the self-evaluation may be intended to give someone else a feel for what's going on in the practice. That person might not be close enough to see the situation, so clarity is essential. When you look at the self-evaluation checklist, be aware that it may be necessary to modify it to fit your hospital; some hospitals may be a bit different and some may be a lot different. Make the checklist as specific as you like.

"If you want someone to understand what you write, write like you speak."

Examples of Self-Evaluation

In this example, I'll evaluate a part of the checklist entitled "Hospital Structure, Leadership, and Management" (Appendix A, section 1.0, p. 89). Within that part and just below it is a bite-sized subsection (1.1) called "Job descriptions in place for each position." First, I'll list the hospital's strengths (Figure 2.1). It's fine to start out on a good note. In listing our strengths, I just use bullet statements. No need to create a long dissertation at this point. The key is to use short, complete thoughts. Now I'll list our weaknesses in this same area (Figure 2.2). Again, short bullet statements will usually suffice. It's important, however, to remember that when listing weaknesses, clarity is critical. A few additional words may be necessary to achieve the level of understanding you desire. Now it's time to write a narrative summary assessment (Figure 2.3).

Figure 2.1 Job descriptions in place for all positions: Strengths

- Technician job descriptions are complete and detailed.
- Pet Lodge job descriptions are complete and detailed.
- Receptionist job descriptions are complete and detailed.

Figure 2.2 Job descriptions in place for all positions: Weaknesses

- Office manager job description is written but not sufficiently detailed.
- Hospital manager job description does not exist.
- Technician assistant job description does not exist.

Figure 2.3 Job descriptions: Assessment

Most of the job descriptions are written for the positions at our hospital. The descriptions are detailed and easily understood. The office manager's job description is written, but several areas were inadvertently left out. The job descriptions for the technician assistant and hospital manager still haven't been written.

Figure 2.4 Doctor average client charge: Strengths

- Dr. Power's ACC is $114.21
- Dr. Okidoki's ACC is $98.47

I'll do another example. Under section 5.5 entitled "Hospital performance" of Appendix A (p. 100), there is an item called "Doctor average client charge (ACC)" (p. 100).

Using the same procedure as before, I'll begin by listing the strengths (Figure 2.4). My responses are short and to the point. Bullet statements are all that are required. The message is clear and understandable. Now I'll list the weaknesses (Figure 2.5). In this instance, listing the weakness in the same manner as the strengths works. The key is to provide the reader with a clear picture of what's happening. Next, I write the assessment in a clear narrative summary (Figure 2.6). The assessment is written as if I was speaking to someone. It tells the

---

Figure 2.5 Doctor average client charge: Weaknesses

- Dr. Donuttin's ACC is $47.90.

Figure 2.6 Doctor average client charge: Assessment

The individual doctor's ACC is generally very good. Two out of three veterinarians are approaching or over $100 ACC. My biggest concern is with Dr. Donuttin. His ACC is less than $50.00. My research indicates that Dr. Donuttin orders virtually no diagnostic tests and he frequently discounts his services for no apparent reason.

---

story clearly. It is tempting to go off on a tangent and tell the reader what I intend to do about the problem. But I won't. The assessment is not the place for that. I simply assessed. Now it's your turn. Try Exercise 2.1.

Exercise 2.1

Using the checklist in Appendix A, find an area where your practice has both good points and bad points. List your strengths, your weaknesses. Then take that information and write an assessment. Remember. Be honest!

Area assessed:

_____

List your strengths:

- _____

- _____

- _____

- _____

List your weaknesses:

- _____

- _____

- _____

- _____

Now pull it all together by writing your assessment. Remember to write like you speak to achieve the greatest degree of clarity.

Assessment: _____

_____

_____

_____

_____

_____

_____

_____

_____

_____

_____

In Exercise 2.2 you will read a scenario and perform a three-part mock self-evaluation.

Exercise 2.2

In the following scenario you'll find everything you need to extract the three parts of the self-evaluation: strengths, weaknesses, and assessment. The scenario will reflect information in the subarea of Key Marketing Functions in Appendix A (section 6.0, p. 102).

Scenario: I have what I consider a progressive small animal clinic. ABC Pet Clinic is located in a major metropolitan area on the fringes of the suburbs. Most of the employees have been with me a long time, but I have noticed a high turnover rate in receptionists over the past year. We computerized the practice 18 months ago. I thought the practice was going to get better once the computers were installed, but business has actually dropped off. We have a fair number of new clients coming through the door, but new customers aren't coming back like they used to. The yellow pages advertisement is very good. Our outside signage is quite large and noticeable. I know reminders are going out because the receptionist who does them told me so. In my strategic business plan, I wrote a good marketing calendar. I delegated the marketing duties to the receptionists. I've thought about putting a referral program together but haven't gotten around to it yet.

Exercise: Look over the part of Appendix A indicated above, analyze the situation, and list the strengths and weakness. Remember to use short bullet statements.

Strengths:

* _____

* _____

* _____

- _____

- _____

Weaknesses:

- _____

- _____

- _____

- _____

- _____

Now, taking the information gathered in the strengths and weaknesses section, write the assessment as a narrative summary.

Assessment: _____

_____

_____

_____

_____

Summary

The important thing to remember about the self-evaluation process is that it is the first step in the strategic and tactical planning process. Diligent, honest appraisals are essential to success. When you get ready to do your self-evaluation, don't allow yourself to be distracted. You may have to do it after hours. I once knew a doctor who hired a relief veterinarian for the day we did the self-evaluation. Systematically work through the list. Take your time and be thorough. Try to get some other people involved. When you've finished, you will feel like you've taken the first step toward curing all that ails your practice—and that you now have a firm grasp on just how your practice is doing. The next step in the strategic planning process is building the action list. As you'll see in the next chapter, action lists provide the crucial link between strategic and tactical plans.

CHAPTER 3

ACTION LISTS

**"If you want action,
you have to use an
action verb."**

In the last chapter, we discussed the self-evaluation part of the strategic plan. We saw that through a detailed self-evaluation you'll discover all the strong points and weak areas of your practice. Now what? What do you do with all this wonderful information? How do you take this information and make it work? The answer to those questions is through action lists.

Defining Action Lists

Simply stated, action lists are the accumulation of all the things you've identified as weaknesses during the self-evaluation process. They also list the goals you aspire to achieve. But action lists are a whole lot more.

At the beginning of the last chapter, we defined the word *strategic* in *strategic plans*: *Necessary to or important in the initiation, conduct or completion of a plan.* This is where action lists come in. An action list will help you initiate and complete your plans and will help you set a timetable for initiating and accomplishing all you want to achieve or accomplish. It will put your plans in a format that is easily used and in fact will become a "living document" that you should place on the top of your desk so it will be easy to find.

Components of Action Lists

It is now appropriate to break down the action list into its components and discuss each. Figure 3.1 (p. 21) is an action list template, and Figure 3.2 (p. 22) is a sample completed action list. The action list template has five main parts arranged as column heads across the page.

- action item
- start date
- completion date
- primary responsibility
- secondary responsibility

That's it. Just those five items round off the process of completing your strategic plan and also set you up to make the transition into tactical plans. For now, let's look at each one of the parts and see how they all fit together.

Action Items

Action items are those things you listed in the self-evaluation as weaknesses. They are also items you may have written out as goals during the self-evaluation process. We have two problems. First, you wrote those weaknesses as short bullet statements. Second, you probably wrote that bullet statement in passive voice. That is to say, the information is matter of fact and just lies there, staring up at you like a recently caught perch.

Let me give you an example. In Figure 2.5 (p. 13), I identified Dr. Donuttin as having a low ACC. I wrote, "Dr. Donuttin's ACC is $47.90." As you can see, the statement only tells you what's wrong. By virtue of their title, action items must be active and must show action. To accomplish this, I will simply rewrite the bullet statement using an action verb: *Train doctors to provide more services.*

Figure 3.1 Action list template

Animal Hospital Name
Company Action List

Action Item	Start Date	Completion Date	Primary Responsibility	Secondary Responsibilty

Figure 3.2 Sample completed action list

Animal Hospital Name
Company Action List

Action Item	Start Date	Completion Date	Primary Responsibility	Secondary Responsibility
1. Ensure rechecks are scheduled	1/1/98	3/31/98	Dr. Okidoki	Brian Hayden
2. Formalize reminder system—written	1/1/98	3/31/98	Michelle Bell	Susan Smith
3. Validate radiation certification	1/1/98	3/31/98	Brian Hayden	Dr. Okidoki
4. Amend radiation log with comments	1/1/98	3/31/98	Brian Hayden	Dana Fargo
5. Initiate chart reviews with doctors	1/1/98	3/31/98	Dr. Okidoki	Brian Hayden
6. Get automatic attendant working properly	1/1/98	3/31/98	Michelle Bell	Henry Potter
7. Establish protocol for estimates	1/1/98	3/31/98	Dr. Okidoki	Dr. Powers
8. Include action plans review at all meetings	1/1/98	3/31/98	Brian Hayden	Dr. Okidoki
9. Develop/implement client service representative (CSR) checklists	1/1/98	2/15/98	Susan Smith	Dr. Okidoki
10. Include mission/vision/values all meetings	1/1/98	1/31/98	Brian Hayden	Dr. Slacks
11. Develop monthly tactical plans/action lists	1/30/98	2/28/98	Brian Hayden	Dr. Okidoki
12. Include financial statement at all meetings	1/30/98	3/31/98	Brian Hayden	Dr. Okidoki
13. Detail each item on general/detail assessment criteria—develop tactical plan to correct. Include on action plan and monthly plans to ensure follow-up	1/30/98	3/31/98	Brian Hayden	Dr. Okidoki

(continues)

Figure 3.2 Sample completed action list (continued)

Animal Hospital Name
Company Action List

	Action Item	Start Date	Completion Date	Primary Responsibility	Secondary Responsibility
14.	Implement customer service training	1/1/98	3/31/98	Susan Smith	Michelle Bell
15.	Develop specific tactical plan to address all training issues	1/1/98	3/15/98	Brian Hayden	Dr. Okidoki
16.	Spotcheck employees—mission/vision	1/1/98	1/31/98	Brian Hayden	Dr. Okidoki
17.	Identify ancillary improvement areas	1/1/98	2/15/98	Brian Hayden	Dr. Okidoki
18.	Initiate methods to make employees accountable	1/19/98	2/15/98	Brian Hayden	Dr. Okidoki
19.	Provide wait-time training	2/1/98	3/31/98	Susan Smith	Michelle Bell
20.	Train employees in angry client management	2/15/98	3/31/98	Susan Smith	Brian Hayden
21.	Train in use of handouts at meetings	2/1/98	3/31/98	Dana Fargo	Susan Smith
22.	Implement hours worked tracking form	2/1/98	2/15/98	All team leaders	Brian Hayden
23.	Get dental special details	1/15/98	1/30/98	Dr. Okidoki	Dr. Pane
24.	Establish referral program	1/20/98	3/30/98	Brian Hayden	Susan Smith
25.	Follow up marketing calendar management meetings	1/20/98	2/1/98	Michelle Bell	Brian Hayden

(continues)

Figure 3.2 Sample completed action list (continued)

Animal Hospital Name
Company Action List

Action Item	Start Date	Completion Date	Primary Responsibility	Secondary Responsibility
26. Develop tactical plan to implement Occupational Safety and Health Administration (OSHA) guidelines	1/30/98	3/30/98	Michelle Bell	Brian Hayden
27. Develop medical records training	2/15/98	6/1/98	Brian Hayden	Marita Brown
28. Update technician duty lists	2/1/98	5/1/98	Brian Hayden	Dr. Okidoki
29. Equipment maintenance use training	2/1/98	5/1/98	Brian Hayden	Dr. Okidoki
30. Develop procedure to reduce missed revenue	2/1/98	4/15/98	Susan Smith	Michelle Bell
31. Clean-up service/inventory codes	1/1/98	4/15/98	Dana Fargo	Lisa Burns
32. Purge all old files from cabinets	1/1/98	3/1/98	Dr. Powers	Dana Fargo
33. Develop leadership trng in meetings	2/1/98	5/30/98	Brian Hayden	Dr. Okidoki
34. Take minutes of meetings, type, distribute	2/1/98	4/1/98	Dr. Okidoki	Brian Hayden
35. Send Susan/Michelle to AAHA management	2/1/98	6/30/98	Susan Smith	Cathy Wise
36. Develop detail job descriptions	4/1/98	6/30/98	Brian Hayden	Dr. Okidoki
37. Plant bushes/flowers in front corner	3/1/98	6/30/98	Michelle Bell	Susan Smith
38. Train/appoint people to run new client letter	2/1/98	4/15/98	Brian Hayden	Dr. Okidoki

(continues)

24

Figure 3.2 Sample completed action list (continued)

Animal Hospital Name
Company Action List

	Action Item	Start Date	Completion Date	Primary Responsibility	Secondary Responsibility
39.	Develop audit for number of phone calls	2/1/98	5/1/98	Dr. Okidoki	Brian Hayden
40.	Monitor on-hold time	2/1/98	4/1/98	Brian Hayden	Dr. Okidoki
41.	Replace air conditioning units	4/1/98	6/1/98	Brian Hayden	Michelle Bell
42.	Train doctors to overcome fee sensitivity	3/1/98	6/1/98	Michelle Bell	Susan Smith
43.	Develop system that better utilizes interns	3/1/98	6/1/98	Susan Smith	Michelle Bell
44.	Develop program to acknowledge top revenue clients	3/1/98	6/1/98	Brian Hayden	Dr. Okidoki
45.	Always offer tours	1/15/98	6/30/98	Dr. Boss	Brian Hayden
46.	Study need for recall programs	1/31/98	6/30/98	Dr. Okidoki	Brian Hayden
47.	Finalize hospital brochures	2/1/98	5/30/98	Dr. Okidoki	Dr. Powers
48.	Develop marketing for Lodge	2/1/98	5/31/98	Dr. Okidoki	Brian Hayden
49.	Develop direct mailer program	3/1/98	6/30/98	all personnel	all personnel
50.	Make logic table regarding air conditioner maintenance versus replacement	3/1/98	5/30/98	Brian Hayden	Dr. Okidoki
51.	Study utilization of space	3/1/98	6/1/98	Dr. Okidoki	Brian Hayden
52.	Develop wellness program marketing	2/1/98	4/1/98	Brian Hayden	Henry Potter

(continues)

Figure 3.2 Sample completed action list (continued)

Animal Hospital Name
Company Action List

	Action Item	Start Date	Completion Date	Primary Responsibility	Secondary Responsibility
53.	Provide anesthetic safety training	5/1/98	8/1/98	Michelle Bell	Brian Hayden
54.	Develop Nosicomial Disease Control	4/1/98	9/1/98	Brian Hayden	Dr. Okidoki
55.	Get outside tower lighted	2/1/98	7/31/98	Brian Hayden	Dr. Okidoki
56.	Send Leo/Dana to AAHA management	7/1/98	9/30/98	Brian Hayden	Dr. Okidoki
57.	Write roles/responsibilities for all employees	6/1/98	9/30/98	Brian Hayden	Dr. Okidoki
58.	Uniform change	8/1/98	9/30/98	Dr. Winters	Marita Brown
59.	Update computers	7/1/98	9/30/98	Dr. Goferit	Dr. Caller
60.	Budget Veterinary Management Institute for Dr. Okidoki/Brian for 1999	10/1/98	12/31/98	Brian Hayden	Dr. Okidoki
61.	Resurface parking lot	10/1/98	12/31/98	Brian Hayden	Dr. Okidoki
62.	Repaint interior walls/cleanable paint	10/1/98	12/31/98	Brian Hayden	Michelle Bell
63.	Replace floor in reception area	10/1/98	12/31/98	Susan Smith	Dr. Okidoki

You can see that by adding an action verb to what's wrong, I converted a passive negative statement to a positive action! Let me give you another example from the previous chapter. In Figure 2.2 (p. 11), I wrote: *Hospital manager job description does not exist.* Again, the statement just lies there. But when I change it around a bit and add an action verb, see what happens: *Write the hospital manager job description.*

Action is what we want. We want to transform all of the issues identified in the self-evaluation into tangible actions that can be accomplished. Here is a list of some action verbs that will prove useful in changing your passive statements into action items.

- develop
- write
- initiate
- compile
- format
- list
- delegate
- train
- coach
- build
- purchase

Of course, there are many more you can use. The important thing is that an action verb sets into motion what you want to accomplish. In Exercise 3.1, you will have an opportunity to create action items.

Exercise 3.1

Using weaknesses you listed in the earlier exercises, change them to action items. Begin by restating the weakness. Then transform it. Do this with at least two items.

Restate weaknesses:

• _____

• _____

• _____

• _____

Transform weakness into action items:

• _____

• _____

• _____

• _____

Action items on a sheet of paper or on a template become your action list. For this part of the planning process, it's not necessary to assign any order to the action items as you place them on the action list. Simply put them on the list in the order you write them. As you'll see later, they will be prioritized when you make your tactical plans.

Start Date

Let's move on to the next part of the action list: the start date. The start date, as the name implies, is the target date on which you want to begin accomplishing that item. There are a couple of rules to follow when you assign start dates in order to avoid pitfalls managers sometimes fall into. My first rule is: Don't try to do everything at once. Many managers I've met assign a start day of, let's say, January 1, 2001, for every item on the action list. That's not realistic. You should use this phase of planning to prioritize the work ahead of you. Start the most important projects first. Perhaps your highest priorities are those that increase the bottom line. Select the action items that will influence the bottom line and assign early start dates to those items. Items that have a lower priority, say, building a shed to store archived records, might be assigned a start date later in the year. You decide what should be done first and what should be done last. Start dates give you the opportunity to look at the big picture of what needs doing and to prioritize your work.

My second rule is: Get people involved in the process of setting the start dates. Every time you involve staff members and get them to agree to a reasonable start date, you've won. You can guide them in setting dates that fit your personal timetable as you allow them to participate and be part of the process.

Completion Date

The third part of the action list is the completion date. Aside from the action item, this is perhaps the most important component. Completion date is the date you expect to complete the action item. There are a number of good reasons you should approach this item with deliberate thought and purpose.

Let me start by saying that those managers who now find themselves in nonmanagerial jobs probably didn't give much thought to setting completion dates for accomplishing the things on their lists. Taking a clue from their experience, you should use the completion date as your opportunity to set a timetable for accomplishing tasks and for clarifying the big picture of your practice. Above all, this is your opportunity to seize success in the planning process.

Just as you wouldn't want to set a goal that couldn't reasonably be reached, you must not set a completion date that cannot be realistically met. We all miss deadlines once in a while. That's just part of life. But setting completion dates that are unrealistic is an exercise that will set you up for disaster. Suppose you set a completion date for December 1, 2000. As the date gets closer, you realize you won't make it. Why does it matter? There are two reasons: First, if you don't finish your project on time, it gets pushed back, which clogs your calendar. You may then become or feel overwhelmed. Instead of reaping the benefits of good planning—a more effective and efficient life—you take a giant step backward when you miss a completion date. Things start to get crazy. Work starts piling up. You and your staff become harried.

Proper planning and date-setting will give you the peace of mind you deserve. Together, a reasonable start date and a realistic completion date will help prioritize your work, spread it out a bit, and allow you to focus on the job at hand. The second consequence of missing a completion date is that you and your staff will miss out on that feeling of accomplishment. There is nothing as motivating and gratifying as bringing in a job on time. Don't miss that opportunity. Give your staff the chance to feel the "win."

Primary Responsibility

The fourth element of the action list is called primary responsibility. As the name implies, in this column of the action list, you name the person who has primary responsibility for accomplishing the item. It's important to keep in mind that planning is a function of management and that other functions of management influence planning. As you go through the planning process, you will need to make a decision: Do I do this task myself or do I delegate the job to someone else?

Most managers I've met have a hard time delegating. For a variety of reasons, they choose to do almost all the tasks themselves. A completed action list shows only the manager's name on the list. May I suggest that you delegate. The goal of planning is to make your system more efficient and to lower your blood pressure. It becomes difficult, if not impossible, to achieve efficiency if you're buried with too much to do. Delegating jobs has many benefits. First, delegating tasks gives you time to do the things you have to do. If you're not overburdened, you can focus on the job at hand. Second, if done correctly, delegating gives your staff a feeling of empowerment. You trusted them to complete a project for the clinic. They are motivated. You benefit twice by getting your staff involved. Conversely, doing all the projects yourself may have adverse effects on the staff. They may develop the feeling that you don't trust them, which may in turn affect their attitudes about their jobs; they may begin to act like they are "just in it for the paycheck." Nobody wants employees like that. Think of yourself as the conductor of an orchestra. Each member of your staff represents a different instrument in the orchestra. If you are going to make the symphony sound right, you have to let all the members of the orchestra play their parts. The concert will not sound very good if you try to play all the parts yourself.

Secondary Responsibility

Secondary responsibility is the final part of the action list. We assign a secondary person to be responsible for accomplishing the action item because good managers always have a contingency plan—

a backup plan if you will. You never know when someone will quit, get sick, or become injured. If there isn't anyone to step in, the project is halted. Additionally, some jobs require the work of more than one person. The person assigned secondary responsibility may also be the extra person assigned to work on the action item. In either case, it is important to list a second person for every task.

Now it's your turn to put together a complete action list (see Exercise 3.2).

Exercise 3.2

Do Exercise 3.2 on the copy of the action list. Use the same information you developed during the earlier exercises. You identified weaknesses and then altered them with an action verb, turning them into action items. Now simply place those action items onto the action list. The order of the items has no bearing at this point. Once the action items are listed, enter the start dates and completion dates. Then assign a person to take primary responsibility. Lastly, assign a person to take secondary responsibility.

Animal Hospital Name
Company Action List

Action Item	Start Date	Completion Date	Secondary Responsibility	Primary Responsibility

Summary

Let's recap the strategic planning process. A strategic plan, the first step in the planning process, defines your goals and identifies the areas that need improvement through the systematic, detailed self-evaluation. After you complete this process, you will have baseline information on where your practice stands today that will enable you to accurately forecast and set attainable goals for the future. Through the self-evaluation, goals will be set, problems identified, and assessments made. The strategic plan draws a picture of your practice, further enabling you and others to understand it. The strategic plan then takes your goals, problems, and projects to an action list, where a timetable for beginning and finishing your action items will be set. People are assigned primary and secondary responsibilities for the projects.

You now have steps for accomplishing your goals and a timetable for helping you keep on track. So with the exception of the budget (which I will not talk about in detail in this book), I think your strategic plan is complete. It's time to kick back, put your feet on the desk, and bask in the glow of a job well done, serene in the knowledge that you just developed a strategic business plan that will carry you gracefully for another year.

Unhappily, if you do so, you would be *wrong!* The total planning process is still a long way from completion. Now is the time for all good managers to come forth and write a tactical business plan.

CHAPTER 4

TACTICAL PLANNING

**❝The best laid plans
of mice and men don't
mean a thing without
a tactical plan!❞**

We have written a great strategic plan. All our goals, aspirations for the practice, trouble spots, and projects have been entered in our action list. Everything seems to be in place. Right? Well, almost. The strategic plan puts the big picture into perspective. It lets you see what's going on and what needs to be done. But there is still the doing left to do. We must find a way to take the information that we gathered in the strategic plan and take the next step, which is, of course, making it happen. Tactical plans make things happen by putting into motion everything outlined in the strategic plan. When I define tactical plans, you will see the link between strategic and tactical plans. You will begin to see that one can't work without the other.

I can't count the number of management seminars, classes, and speeches I've attended over the past 25 years. Thinking back on them, I don't believe I've ever heard a single syllable about tactical plans. There was plenty of discussion about strategic plans. Perhaps if the speakers had written a tactical plan to address the issues of planning, they wouldn't have forgotten to discuss them!

Tactical plans aren't a commodity. You can't go to the local store and pick a plan off the shelf. You must select the type of tactical plan that meets the needs of the scenario presented, which requires a certain degree of knowledge on your part. I'll begin by introducing you to the various types of tactical plans, explaining what each one is used for, and defining the tactical planning process. Then we'll examine each type of plan individually, look at its parts, and learn how to use it.

> **❝Working a defined process is much easier than defining the process as you work.❞**

Types of Tactical Plans

A tactical plan will transform your action list into a tool that will help you to stay on track as you do the things that need doing. To understand the tactical planning process, you need to agree that the purpose of the process is to break down and organize the information in your strategic plan.

To begin the process of breaking down the strategic plan, we have two primary types of tactical plans. They are, as you might have guessed, based on time. Their purpose again is to help you get the jobs done in the time frame you've laid out in the strategic plan. The plans are called *quarterly master action plans* and *monthly tactical action plans*. Although we'll be discussing them in separate chapters in more detail later, let's briefly look at each one and see how they fit into the total planning process.

Quarterly Master Action Plans

The quarterly master action plan (QMAP) is the first line of tactical plans. That is to say, a QMAP is the first transitional tool you use to go from the strategic plan to the tactical plan. The QMAP will put your action items in a format that will help you keep track of them. It will assist you in accomplishing your objectives in the timetable you have specified. With all your action items in hand, sort them by estimated completion dates. Then begin plugging them into the QMAP. Put the items you expect to complete in the first quarter in the area of the QMAP entitled *First Quarter*. It's really quite simple. I'll go more into detail about QMAPs and how to use them later. At this point it is important to recognize that a QMAP is a valuable tactical tool that will help you immensely in staying on track and accomplishing everything you want.

Monthly Tactical Action Plans

The second type of tactical plan is called a monthly tactical action plan (MTAP). Remember the advice at the beginning of Chapter 2 about eating an elephant one bite at a time. This is the next logical step in breaking down the big picture—namely, strategic plans and quarterly master action plans—into smaller, easier-to-accomplish steps (or bites). The whole planning process is a method of taking the big picture and methodically breaking it down to a manageable size. As you continue in the process, you come to the last step: the MTAP. It is, as they say, where the tires hit the road. This part actually makes things happen.

We use two types of MTAPs: grocery lists and comprehensive plans. Let's briefly look at each. Tactical plans—like grocery lists—keep us on track by simply listing the things that need to be done. I use them for both monthly and daily tasks. The second type of MTAP is the comprehensive plan. Do you recall the story about the dental special? Complex projects that require a multifaceted approach require a comprehensive plan. Had I done one, my dental special would have gone off without a hitch and without the confusion and frustration that accompanied it. Comprehensive plans are critical to the success of singular complex projects.

Definition of Tactical Plans

Let's define tactical plans so we are sure we understand their meaning. Earlier in the book, we discussed the definition of strategic plans and we saw that the adjective in front of the word *plan* distinguishes the type of plan we're using. Let's review the definition of *plans*.

- A method for achieving an end
- A detailed formulation of a program of action
- Goal, aim
- An orderly arrangement of parts of an overall design or objective

Even when we talk about tactical plans, we're still just talking about plans. We only really need to figure out what the *tactical* part means. The dictionary gives us about fifteen or so definitions, of which about four apply.

- Of or relating to small-scale actions serving a larger purpose
- Made, or carried out, with only a limited or immediate end in view
- Adept in planning or maneuvering to accomplish a purpose
- Of or relating to management or order

The definition of *tactical* tells us that we're dealing with the small picture, the basic component of what we want. It defines tactical as relating to a short-term project with a definite end in sight and a specific step-by-step procedure for accomplishing a goal or task. Lastly, and quite profoundly, the definition tells us that "tactics" are fundamental tools managers use to maintain order or to keep things organized. We can see that a tactical plan is one we can use to get the job done!

We'll now look again at the types of tactical plans and we'll apply the definitions. Then you will see the power of tactical plans. You will be able to understand the planning process and how each step along the way leads to the next.

CHAPTER 5

QUARTERLY MASTER ACTION PLANS

*"To err is human,
but failing to properly plan
is just asking for trouble."*

From time to time, you may think that passages of this book are redundant. You are right! For many of you, a formal planning process is new. Although you've planned things in the past, you may not have used a structured, detailed planning process that takes you from the big picture right down to the smallest detail and finishes the job. My method of explanation is a building-block process. Some of you who read this book and who have had formal training in planning may find my approach a bit different from the one you are used to. There are many planning processes. I urge you, however, to try my step-by-step process and see how effective it is.

The Importance of Quarterly Master Action Plans

Let's focus on quarterly master action plans (QMAPs). As I mentioned earlier, QMAPs are the first step in making the transition from strategic plans to tactical plans. In other words, the QMAP takes the vision of what you want to accomplish and begins to break it down to the point that goals can be accomplished, tasks can be completed, and progress can be measured. Just as tactical plans come directly from strategic plans, a QMAP takes the information directly from the action list prepared in the strategic plan and organizes it in a way that helps you accomplish things.

If you look at the example of a QMAP in Figure 5.1, you will find that the layout is almost identical to that of the action list. That is because we want to establish a direct link back to strategic plans. If you don't establish a direct link back to the previous step in the process, the planning process won't be going forward in the direction the strategic plans laid out for us. It'll wind up going in a haphazard fashion, without regard for the big picture. So the direct link to the strategic plan is critical!

Effecting the Transition

The way we effect the transition from the action list (strategic plan) and the QMAP (tactical plan) is by grouping our goals, objectives, and projects into periods of time (i.e., by calendar quarter). If you look at the action list you completed earlier, you will recall that all the things listed were simply put into the format as they were identified through the self-evaluation process. Beginning dates and completion dates were established, but they weren't listed by date on the action list. On the QMAP, we'll sort our action list items by completion dates. Once that is done, just plug the items into the QMAP according to the quarter in which it is to be completed. Because the format of the QMAP is virtually identical to that of an action list, no additional work is needed. This part of the process will organize the things you want to get done in chronological order by calendar quarter.

To get a feel for what I am talking about, take all those action items we identified and listed in the action list earlier and put them into the QMAP provided. (You may want to make some copies of the blank format offered in Figure 5.2 to use in your own practice.)

I've provided four different blank QMAPs. The only difference between them is that they are marked on the top: 1st quarter, 2nd quarter, and so on. When you use these blanks in your practice, enter

Figure 5.1 Sample Quarterly Master Action Plan

Animal Hospital Name
Quarterly Master Action Plan

Action Item	Start Date	Completion Date	Primary Responsibility	Secondary Responsibility	Status
1st Quarter '98					
1. Ensure rechecks are scheduled	1/1/98	3/31/98	Dr. Okidoki	Brian Hayden	
2. Formalize reminder system—written	1/1/98	3/31/98	Michelle Bell	Susan Smith	
3. Validate radiation certification	1/1/98	3/31/98	Brian Hayden	Dr. Okidoki	
4. Amend radiation log with comments	1/1/98	3/31/98	Brian Hayden	Dana Fargo	
5. Initiate chart reviews with doctors	1/1/98	3/31/98	Dr. Okidoki	Brian Hayden	
6. Get automatic attendant working properly	1/1/98	3/31/98	Michelle Bell	Henry Potter	
7. Establish protocol for estimates	1/1/98	3/31/98	Dr. Clark	Dr. Powers	
8. Include action plans review at all meetings	1/1/98	1/31/98	Brian Hayden	Dr. Okidoki	
9. Develop/implement CSR checklists	1/1/98	3/15/98	Susan Smith	Dr. Okidoki	
10. Include mission/vision/values at all meetings	1/1/98	1/31/98	Brian Hayden	Dr. Slacks	
11. Develop monthly tactical plans/action	1/30/98	2/28/98	Brian Hayden	Dr. Okidoki	
12. Include financial statement at all meetings	1/30/98	3/31/98	Brian Hayden	Dr. Okidoki	
13. Detail each item on general/detail assessment criteria—develop tactical plan to correct. Include on action plan and monthly plans to ensure follow-up	1/30/98	3/31/98	Brian Hayden	Dr. Okidoki	

(continues)

Figure 5.1 Sample Quarterly Master Action Plan (continued)

Animal Hospital Name
Quarterly Master Action Plan

Action Item	Start Date	Completion Date	Primary Responsibility	Secondary Responsibility	Status
14. Implement customer service training	1/1/98	3/31/98	Susan Smith	Michelle Bell	
15. Develop specific tactical plan to address all training issues	1/1/98	3/15/98	Brian Hayden	Dr. Okidoki	
16. Spotcheck employees—mission/vision	1/1/98	1/31/98	Brian Hayden	Dr. Okidoki	
17. Identify ancillary improvement areas	1/1/98	2/15/98	Brian Hayden	Dr. Okidoki	
18. Initiate methods to make employees accountable	1/19/98	2/15/98	Brian Hayden	Dr. Okidoki	
19. Provide wait-time training	2/1/98	3/31/98	Susan Smith	Michelle Bell	
20. Train employees in angry client management	2/15/98	3/31/98	Susan Smith	Brian Hayden	
21. Train in use of handouts at meetings	2/1/98	3/31/98	Dana Fargo	Susan Smith	
22. Implement hours worked tracking form	2/1/98	2/15/98	All team leaders	Brian Hayden	
23. Get dental special details	1/15/98	1/30/98	Dr. Okidoki	Dr. Pane	
24. Establish referral program	1/20/98	3/30/98	Brian Hayden	Susan Smith	
25. Follow up marketing calendar management meetings	1/20/98	2/1/98	Michelle Bell	Brian Hayden	
26. Develop tactical plan to implement OSHA guidelines	1/30/98	3/30/98	Brian Hayden	Marita Brown	

(continues)

Figure 5.1 Sample Quarterly Master Action Plan (continued)

Animal Hospital Name
Quarterly Master Action Plan

Action Item	Start Date	Completion Date	Primary Responsibility	Secondary Responsibility	Status
2nd Quarter '98					
1. Develop medical records training	2/15/98	6/1/98	Susan Smith	Michelle Bell	
2. Update technician duty lists	2/1/98	5/1/98	Dana Fargo	Lisa Burns	
3. Equipment maintenance/use training	2/1/98	5/1/98	Dr. Powers	Dana Fargo	
4. Develop procedure to reduce missed revenue	2/1/98	4/15/98	Brian Hayden	Dr. Okidoki	
5. Clean-up service/inventory codes	1/1/98	4/15/98	Dr. Okidoki	Brian Hayden	
6. Purge all old files from cabinets	1/1/98	3/1/98	Susan Smith	Cathy Wise	
7. Develop leadership trng in meetings	2/1/98	5/30/98	Brian Hayden	Dr. Okidoki	
8. Take minutes of meetings, type, and distribute	2/1/98	4/1/98	Michelle Bell	Susan Smith	
9. Send Susan/Michelle to AAHA management	2/1/98	6/30/98	Brian Hayden	Dr. Okidoki	
10. Develop detail job descriptions	4/1/98	6/30/98	Brian Hayden	Dr. Okidoki	
11. Plant bushes/flowers in front corner	3/1/98	6/30/98	Brian Hayden	Michelle Bell	
12. Train/appoint people to run new client letter	2/1/98	4/15/98	Michelle Bell	Susan Smith	
13. Develop audit for number of phone calls	2/1/98	5/1/98	Susan Smith	Michelle Bell	
14. Monitor on-hold time	2/1/98	4/1/98	Brian Hayden	Dr. Okidoki	

(continues)

Figure 5.1 Sample Quarterly Master Action Plan (continued)

Animal Hospital Name
Quarterly Master Action Plan

	Action Item	Start Date	Completion Date	Primary Responsibility	Secondary Responsibility	Status
15.	Replace air conditioning units	4/1/98	6/1/98	Dr. Boss	Brian Hayden	
16.	Train doctors to overcome fee sensitivity	3/1/98	6/1/98	Dr. Okidoki	Brian Hayden	
17.	Develop system that better utilizes interns	3/1/98	6/1/98	Dr. Okidoki	Dr. Powers	
18.	Develop program to acknowledge top dollar clients	3/1/98	6/1/98	Dr. Okidoki	Brian Hayden	
19.	Always offer tours	1/15/98	6/30/98	all personnel	all personnel	
20.	Study need for recall programs	1/31/98	6/30/98	Brian Hayden	Dr. Okidoki	
21.	Finalize hospital brochures	2/1/98	5/30/98	Dr. Okidoki	Brian Hayden	
22.	Develop marketing for Lodge	2/1/98	5/31/98	Brian Hayden	Henry Potter	
23.	Develop direct mailer program	3/1/98	6/30/98	Michelle Bell	Brian Hayden	
24.	Make logic table regarding air conditioner maintenance versus replacement	3/1/98	5/30/98	Brian Hayden	Dr. Okidoki	
25.	Study utilization of space	3/1/98	6/1/98	Brian Hayden	Dr. Okidoki	
26.	Develop wellness program marketing	2/1/98	4/1/98	Michelle Bell	Dr. Okidoki	

(continues)

Figure 5.1 Sample Quarterly Master Action Plan (continued)

Animal Hospital Name
Quarterly Master Action Plan

Action Item	Start Date	Completion Date	Primary Responsibility	Secondary Responsibility	Status
3rd Quarter '98					
1. Provide anesthetic safety training	5/1/98	8/1/98	Dr. Winters	Marita Brown	
2. Develop Nosicomial Disease Control	4/1/98	9/1/98	Dr. Goferit	Dr. Caller	
3. Get outside tower lighted	2/1/98	7/31/98	Brian Hayden	Dr. Okidoki	
4. Send Leo/Dana to AAHA management	7/1/98	9/30/98	Brian Hayden	Dr. Okidoki	
5. Write roles/responsibilities for all employees	6/1/98	9/30/98	Brian Hayden	Michelle Bell	
6. Uniform change	8/1/98	9/30/98	Susan Smith	Dr. Okidoki	
7. Update computers	7/1/98	9/30/98	Brian Hayden	Dr. Okidoki	
4th Quarter '98					
1. Budget Veterinary Management Institute for Dr. Okidoki/Brian for 1999	10/1/98	12/31/98	Brian Hayden	Dr. Okidoki	
2. Resurface parking lot	10/1/98	12/31/98	Brian Hayden	Dr. Okidoki	
3. Repaint interior walls/cleanable paint	10/1/98	12/31/98	Brian Hayden	Dr. Okidoki	
4. Replace floor in reception area	10/1/98	12/31/98	Brian Hayden	Dr. Okidoki	

Figure 5.2 Sample blank quarterly master action plan

Animal Hospital Name
Quarterly Master Action Plan, First Quarter

Action Item	Start Date	Completion Date	Primary Responsibility	Secondary Responsibility	Status

(continues)

Figure 5.2 Sample blank quarterly master action plan (continued)

Animal Hospital Name
Quarterly Master Action Plan, Second Quarter

Action Item	Start Date	Completion Date	Primary Responsibility	Secondary Responsibility	Status

(continues)

Figure 5.2 Sample blank quarterly master action plan (continued)

Animal Hospital Name
Quarterly Master Action Plan, Third Quarter

Action Item	Start Date	Completion Date	Primary Responsibility	Secondary Responsibility	Status

(continues)

Figure 5.2 Sample blank quarterly master action plan (continued)

Animal Hospital Name
Quarterly Master Action Plan, Fourth Quarter

Action Item	Start Date	Completion Date	Primary Responsibility	Secondary Responsibility	Status

the calendar dates that apply. It is important to note that this QMAP format won't change from practice to practice. From small clinics to huge medical centers, the format remains the same. The only difference might be in the number of pages needed to list the issues. Obviously, the larger the practice, the more action items there will be. Consequently, more pages for the QMAP will be needed.

Exercise 5.1 should give you practice in how a QMAP organizes the work that needs to be done.

Exercise 5.1

In the following scenario, I've listed some items and put them in an action list format. Put those items into the QMAP.

- *Develop training for technicians; Start date: 2/1/99; Completion date: 6/30/99; Primary responsibility: Joe Smith; Secondary responsibility: Mary Jones*
- *Paint exam room 1: Start date: 2/1/99; Completion date: 2/15/99; Primary responsibility: Harry Mutts; Secondary responsibility: Bob Bones*
- *Develop referral program: Start date: 11/1/99; Completion date: 2/15/2000; Primary responsibility: Jane Smarty; Secondary responsibility: Schmoopy Mills*
- *Provide exam room training for doctors: Start date: 1/1/99; Completion date: 1/30/99; Primary responsibility: Dr. Power; Secondary responsibility: Dr. Okidoki*
- *Write employee handbook: Start date: 6/1/99; Completion date: 2/15/2000; Primary responsibility: Dr. Boss; Secondary responsibility: Mary Manager*

As you can see, when you take the information from the action list and put it in the QMAP, your work stands out, prioritized and ready to be completed. The acronym is quite appropriate because the QMAP is a map of the things you want to accomplish throughout the year. It will guide you and remind you from one month to the next. If you keep it on your desk and use it, the QMAP will keep you on the straight and narrow road until you complete everything you wanted to do.

"If you say you'll have it done in April, it must be entered in the second quarter."

CHAPTER 6

MONTHLY TACTICAL ACTION PLANS

"A penny for your thoughts is still a penny, but monthly tactical action plans are priceless."

We've taken our planning process from the big picture in strategic plans, laid out our goals for the year in our action lists, made the transition into tactical plans, prioritizing our work and further clarifying when we want to do things with the quarterly master action plans. But there is still something missing: We haven't actually done any work yet! To make sure we get the work done in a timely manner, we need to take the information we put together in the QMAP and bring it closer to the working level. To provide this transition, the monthly tactical action plan (MTAP) is required.

The Importance of the Monthly Tactical Action Plan

The monthly tactical action plan is used to keep you on track in your month-to-month and day-to-day activities. The MTAP will ensure that things that need to be done are accomplished. It will help keep you organized. And when your work is organized, you become more effective, more efficient, and subsequently more productive. When you are more productive, you become more profitable! And that's what planning is all about. After all, if you can't affect the bottom line in some way, why bother?

Types of Monthly Tactical Action Plans

In the tactical planning process, there are essentially two types of MTAPs: grocery lists and comprehensive plans.

> ❝OK, honey, just write
> it down so I won't
> forget something.❞

Grocery Lists

Grocery lists are perhaps your most flexible tool for making sure things get accomplished. Many of you already use them. You just don't call them grocery lists. A grocery list simply lists all the things you want to accomplish in any given period of time. As you can imagine, there may be a lot of things that will be started or completed in any given month. You start by looking at the QMAPs. A few days before the end of the month, I find those items that should be started in the upcoming month. I simply enter those items on my list without regard for priority. Once I have all the items written in my monthly grocery list, I look back to the month that's about to end. I identify any items that for some reason didn't get completed and bring those items forward to the next month.

A grocery list can help you prioritize your work either daily, weekly, or monthly. Once the list is completed, write down a number to the left of each project that prioritizes your work. That way you can get the most important things done first. When you've finished, you have a neat, prioritized list that will maintain the course and show you how you are progressing.

Grocery lists will keep you from forgetting things. You know how easy it can be to get sidetracked with an emergency or some other crisis. When you finally get back to your desk, you've forgotten what you were doing. Grocery lists will remind you. They are used primarily as monthly and daily lists, but can be used as weekly lists too, depending on how much there is to do and how big an operation you have. Naturally, the bigger the practice, the more things will need to be done. So the time interval for a list is a personal choice. However frequently you make your list, use it in a way that will best keep you on track for getting things done and in a way that fits your personal management style. In Figure 6.1, I've created a typical monthly grocery list; it is much shorter than usual—my lists often have 30 or more items on them. But I run large facilities. In smaller places, the list might be smaller.

Appendix B, Top 300 Things to Do, may be of help to you in creating your grocery list. I'm sure I omitted some items, but my list will help you to remember to include a variety of things you want to accomplish on a daily, weekly, or monthly grocery list. You will also notice that my top 300 list includes tasks that other people will do. As

---

Figure 6.1 Sample monthly grocery list

January

- Begin writing employee manual
- Get paint for exam rooms and schedule work
- Analyze end-of-the-month reports
- Get estimates for kennel renovations
- Prepare meeting agenda
- Complete doctor training
- Write hospital manager job description
- Develop details for dental special

the manager, you'll have to follow up on many projects and jobs that are being done at your hospital. If it's your job to check and make sure the job gets done, put it on your grocery list.

See how helpful a grocery list can be. Even if you do get pulled off in another direction, the grocery list will be there to get you back on track. It won't let you forget! Just be sure that your list includes everything you want to do during the month. You can practice creating a grocery list in Exercise 6.1.

Exercise 6.1

Using a typical month in the life of your practice, build a monthly grocery list. Be sure to include projects that you want to start this month as well as those that must be completed. Once you've written the list, go back through it and determine the priority for completing the tasks listed. This is an excellent time to really manage your workload and become more productive. Get the most important jobs done first.

March Grocery List

- _____

- _____

- _____

- _____

- _____

- _____

- _____

- _____

- _____

You are now ready to try Exercise 6.2.

Exercise 6.2

Now take the QMAP you wrote earlier and put that into a MTAP format. For our purposes here, use all of the examples. Think of half of them as starting in February and the rest as being completed in February. Although there are no right or wrong answers in terms of prioritizing the lists, look over the list you compiled and prioritize the items on the list.

February Grocery List

- _____

- _____

- _____

- _____

- _____

- _____

- _____

- _____

- _____

- _____

- _____

Weekly grocery lists are the same as monthly ones, but they break down the workload for you into smaller, bite-sized pieces. The daily lists, however, warrant a brief discussion. It's by using your daily lists that the work can actually be managed. As you are well aware, new and different situations arise all the time. In the daily lists, you get the flexibility to adjust to the situation at hand. Flexibility is crucial in maintaining order and focus to see the job through. Again, productivity is affected in a positive way—and when you are producing efficiently, your profit increases. As managers, we must continuously adjust our daily schedules to account for variations in what we thought was going to happen. We follow up on the work others are doing and a thousand other details that are thrown in the mix. Without daily lists to keep us focused, all sorts of things would fall through the cracks. Remember that it's the manager's job to make certain every task that must be done gets completed on time. If we fail, we are remiss in our responsibilities to the practice. Daily lists will help you immensely in the completion of goals, tasks, and issues that need to be addressed on a daily basis.

As with monthly lists, daily lists also provide a platform for you to prioritize your daily workload. Use the same system for the daily lists as you did in the monthly ones. See Figure 6.2 for an example of a typical daily list. As you can see, it simply enumerates what must be done that day. Daily lists, used in conjunction with the other grocery lists, are a key element to the overall planning process. Getting in the habit of using grocery lists will go a very long way in helping you achieve success and maintaining control of your practice.

There is one other interesting point about grocery lists that you may already have noticed. All MTAPs, whether daily, weekly, or monthly, need to be written using the active voice and action verbs. Use the same verbs we discussed earlier.

Figure 6.2 Sample daily grocery list

Tuesday

- Contact contractors to get bid on painting room
- Review daily reports from yesterday
- Write vacation part of employee manual
- Write agenda for this afternoon's staff meeting
- Follow up with Mary on progress for her action list items
- Get details together for dental special—add to meeting agenda

The Comprehensive Monthly Tactical Action Plan

The next type of monthly tactical action plan is called the comprehensive plan. As you may have guessed, although it is in the same category as the grocery list (i.e., monthly tactical action plans), the nature of the comprehensive plan is totally different. Until now, we have been talking about lists that encompass a variety of tasks or action items. We looked at the big picture—a whole year's view in our strategic plan—to the smaller picture—the daily grocery lists. With comprehensive plans, we will take a single action item and develop a plan to ensure its successful completion.

Although it may seem that we are simply creating paperwork, I know that if I had completed a comprehensive plan for my dental special, I wouldn't have wasted an entire day trying to fix the problem. Not planning properly cost me an entire day's productivity. Everything I was going to do was pushed back at least a day, which, in turn, jammed up other days, and it was weeks before I caught up. That whole issue not only lost productive time but put a great deal of stress on me for weeks.

The whole idea of implementing the total planning process is to keep you productive, keep you profitable, and minimize stress. This part of the process, if used properly, will do all those things for you. You can't be productive if you're busy running here and there putting out fires. And you can't maximize your profitability if you are not staying productive! Proper planning is so well meshed with everything we do in day-to-day hospital operations that without it, the bottom line will ultimately suffer. The comprehensive plan is just another piece of the total planning process.

> **❝Knowledge is power: the more you know, the more powerful your result.❞**

Knowledge Is Power

That statement is so true. I believe that a manager at any level who is trying to manage any function in a hospital and lacks even some of the information needed is destined to fail. You can't complete the job if you don't know *all* the details associated with it. Managers must have every bit of information available to properly manage their hospitals. This information, unfortunately, does not magically appear on our desks overnight, like the tooth fairy delivering a dollar. We must find it. We must develop it.

We must sometimes get other people involved to obtain information. We must do whatever is necessary to get all the tools we need to get a job done. In other words, we must develop comprehensive plans. Comprehensive plans are developed to provide information about a single project. It's not enough to say you want to do something, say, have a dental special. To successfully complete a project you have to answer some very important questions. But before I get too far ahead of myself, let's define the comprehensive plan.

Definition of a Comprehensive Plan

Like the other terms we've been discussing, comprehensive plans are simply plans. The adjective *comprehensive* describes the type of plan we're using. I define *comprehensive* as "all encompassing," "total or complete." A comprehensive plan provides us with all the information necessary to manage and produce effective results in the implementation of a single project.

> **"You can't do a job justice if you just don't have all the information."**

Information Gathering

Gathering detailed information is the cornerstone of this type of plan. The information-gathering process may, at times, be very time consuming and difficult. You, however, have the power to make it easier by getting your staff involved. In a nutshell, this process should be a group effort. Sit down with at least two or three of the principal players who will be responsible for implementing or actually working the project. They will undoubtedly come up with ideas, suggestions, and pieces of the puzzle that you alone may rack your brains about for hours and still not think of. Don't underestimate the abilities of your staff—especially when it comes to providing you with new and fresh ideas for making your practice work better. Give them the opportunity to participate and you'll receive a payoff in ways you can't even imagine. Given the chance, your employees will provide innovative approaches to problem solving, new concepts in marketing, and many other cost-cutting and money-making ideas.

When Do You Know a Project Needs a Comprehensive Plan?

To determine if a project needs a comprehensive plan, first look at your QMAP. Scan ahead at least one quarter beyond where you are now. As you look through the projects and goals you've written down, pick any single item on the list and ask yourself this: "Is there any other information that I need to know to complete this project?" If the answer is "Yes," a comprehensive plan is probably in order.

What Category Will Your Project Fall Into?

Ultimately, all projects will fall into one of two categories: Either they will be listed on a grocery list or they will require a comprehensive plan to successfully be completed. Let me give you an example. Suppose you run across an item on your QMAP that says, "Write the hospital manager job description." What will it take for you to write the job description? A pen and a piece of paper. You might also pull out some sample job descriptions you've accumulated over the years. That's it. All that really needs to be done is the doin'.

Now compare that task to that darn dental special. I have to outline what the special will consist of, when it will take place, any marketing schemes that will be used and when they will be used, develop a method for tracking its success and make sure that it is in place prior to the start of the special. Additionally, the veterinarians and the staff must be briefed in advance of the special so they can sell it and work it in the way you've outlined. Extra supplies may need to be ordered, the work schedule may need to be altered, and budgets may need to be adjusted.

Multitasking Projects

I call this sort of project, which has many facets—lots of issues that must be addressed and coordinated within a timetable in order to ensure success—a multitasking project. When you are faced with developing and completing multitasking projects, the comprehensive plan will prove invaluable (Exercise 6.3).

Exercise 6.3

List five projects best accomplished through a comprehensive plan.

- _____

- _____

- _____

- _____

- _____

Now list five projects for which a grocery list will suffice.

- _____

- _____

- _____

- _____

- _____

Comparing the lists you wrote, can you see the differences between comprehensive plan items and grocery list items?

It's important to realize that parts of the comprehensive plans may, from time to time, show up on grocery lists. You may already have seen evidence of that when I said that I would work on parts of my dental special on a daily grocery list. Comprehensive plans lay out the entire project; your grocery lists define for you what must be done in a given period of time. Thus, we can say that grocery lists are focused on time and initiation of work, while comprehensive plans are focused on development and completion of work. Together, they help complete the planning process and assist you in running your hospital efficiently.

How Do You Know When You Need a Comprehensive Plan?

When you start asking yourself the following questions, you know you must write a comprehensive plan.

- When does the project need to be finished?
- Who is going to do it?
- What specifically needs to be done?
- When does each part of the project need to be completed?
- Who will do each part?
- Do we need to track it?
- How much will it cost?

Depending on the project, many other issues and questions will need to be settled.

How Do You Build a Comprehensive Plan?

You might be asking yourself, "What format do I use?" "How do I write a plan like this?" Here is a six-step guide to building a comprehensive plan.

Step 1: Brainstorming for questions. If you think about the result you are looking for in writing a comprehensive plan, the format becomes clear. The result is to outline the steps and functions of a single project. The key word is outline. Comprehensive plans are outlines written in a seminarrative format. There is some preliminary work that will need to be done, however, before comprehensive plans can be written. Gather your group together and begin thinking of questions about the project that will need to be answered. Don't be critical of the questions at this point; just write down everything people say.

Step 2: Reviewing questions for applicability. Begin going over each question and evaluate it for relevance. Ask the group, "Does this question have an impact on the project? Yes or no?" If the answer is yes, include it in your comprehensive plan. If the answer is no, discard that question. Let me give you an example. Suppose you had a project on the table for developing a veterinary technician-training program. The following questions might be posed during a brainstorming session.

- What topics will be taught?
- How long will each section be?
- Who will teach each section?
- Will there be tests?
- Who will write the various sections?
- How much time will we devote to writing the training program?
- Will people get raises if they pass the training program?

Looking at the list of questions, can you tell which question has no relevance to accomplishing this project? If you selected the last question concerning raises, you would have been right. All of the other questions have a direct impact on accomplishing this project. They must be answered. Only the question about raises has no bearing on the completion of this task. It's true, of course, that this question will need to be answered somewhere down the road, but it will become a matter of policy as opposed to a step in the procedure for completing the project.

Now that you've weeded out the irrelevant questions (the questions that have no bearing on the process of completing the project), you are ready to move into the heart of the matter: writing the comprehensive plan.

Step 3: Writing the comprehensive plan. This part of the process is simple. Begin by assigning a number to each of the questions that remain after the weeding out process is complete. At this point, it really doesn't matter which questions get which numbers. The list that results from the questions I developed in the last scenario about training should look like this:

1. What topics will be taught?
2. How long will each section be?
3. Who will teach each section?
4. Will there be tests?
5. Who will write the various sections?
6. How much time will we devote to writing the training program?

This list becomes the skeleton for your outline. Everything else will be filled within each numbered topic.

Step 4: Filling out each numbered section. The next step, as you might have guessed, is filling in each numbered section.

> **❝If you intend to write an outline, write an outline, not a book.❞**

Just a short note about this next step: Keep it brief. Say what you must for clarity's sake, but no more. More is not necessarily better. In the following example, I'll break down item number 1.

What topics will be taught?

1a. Placing catheters
1b. Inducing anesthetics
1c. Reading electrocardiograms: the most common problems
1d. Preparing for most common surgeries
1e. Monitoring vitals during anesthetic procedures
1f. Radiographic placement and technique
1g. Administering fluids
1h. Calculating dose rates
1i. Operating computerized lab equipment
1j. Entering hospital charges in the computer
1k. Maintaining patient records
1l. Maintaining equipment

I could continue to list many other items on this topic. I think you can see, however, that at this point in the development of the outline, we must be specific. This step is an excellent opportunity for getting your staff involved. Although some of the projects you will write plans for may not be so in-depth or complex, when you do have topics such as training to write about, the more minds on the job, the better the outcome. Exercise 6.4 gives you an opportunity to break down the remaining questions on our list.

Exercise 6.4

Using the numbered list of questions above, break down numbers two, three, four, and five. Draw the topics for the breakdown process from your hospital environment.

- _____

- _____

- _____

- _____

- _____

- _____

- _____

- _____

- _____

Depending on your hospital's mission, environment, and other factors, each list will be different. The list for large hospitals with emergency equipment and critical care facilities will look dramatically different from the list for a veterinary clinic whose forte is wellness programs and community health. Comprehensive plans are supposed to be flexible enough to accommodate any situation. All hospitals, regardless of their size, will benefit from them.

Step 5: Reevaluating topics. Once you've broken down each numbered section into the main topics (that is, into the main areas of concern within each of the sections), it's time once again for evaluation. Look at each section separately and evaluate the need for further breakdown. Not every topic will require further breakdown—only those areas that have multiple subtopics. For example, I broke down the first question (What topics will be taught?) into subtopics. The first subtopic I listed was "placing catheters." Figure 6.3 demonstrates how to break that subtopic down even further. By breaking the topic down one level at a time, you can systematically create your project in an outline format. Remember, though, each topic will have different levels of structure. This particular topic (training) has a great deal of depth—more than I have addressed in the examples and the exercises. In addition, each hospital will have its own requirements, so this part of the process may be quite different from one hospital to another.

Figure 6.3 Subtopic breakdown

I. What topics will be taught?
    1. placing catheters
        a. venous catheters
            1) jugular (dog/cat)
            2) cephalic (dog/cat)
            3) saphenous (dog/cat)
        b. urinary catheters
            1) dogs (male/female)
            2) cats (male/female)

Apply this principle to Exercise 6.5

Exercise 6.5

Using your answers to Exercise 6.4, break them down into the final level. Remember, not all topics must be broken down. Only break down the topic if doing so achieves greater clarity of purpose. If you already achieved the clarity desired, don't go any further.

- _____

- _____

- _____

- _____

- _____

- _____

Step 6: Finishing the plan. We have almost completed the comprehensive plan. The final step is to clarify what we want to accomplish by fleshing out the items verbally. We begin with Figure 6.3, and by turning the outline vocabulary into more complete sentences and phrases, we finalize the comprehensive plan (see Figure 6.4). As you can see, I didn't add too much—just enough to clarify my outline. Notice, also, I didn't go off on a tangent and discuss how the material would be taught, how long it will take, or who would do the training. Those issues are addressed in other areas of the comprehensive plan. Here I wanted to focus on the original issue: "What topics will be taught?" Complete a portion of the comprehensive plan in Exercise 6.6.

Figure 6.4 Completed subtopic breakdown of comprehensive plan

Venous catheters: Veterinary technicians must display a proficiency in placing the following types of venous catheters:

- jugular (dogs and cats)
- cephalic (dogs and cats)
- saphenous (dogs and cats)

Urinary catheters: Veterinary technicians must display proficiency in placing both tomcat and Foley catheters and knowing which is appropriate to use.

- dogs (male and female)
- cats (male and female)

Exercise 6.6

Select two topics you outlined in Exercise 6.5. Rewrite the outline as a filled-in narrative description of that part of the comprehensive plan.

_____

_____

_____

_____

_____

_____

_____

_____

_____

_____

This process isn't too time-consuming or difficult, especially if it is done as a group effort. And the effort will be well worth it when you get ready to start a project on your QMAP. Try your hand on the final exercise (Exercise 6.7).

Exercise 6.7

Take an action item from the QMAP, which addresses issues in your own hospital. Write a comprehensive plan based on your hospital's reality.

_____

_____

_____

_____

_____

_____

_____

_____

_____

Summary

If done correctly, comprehensive plans make your life easier, less stressful, and more profitable. Never again will you be working on a project only to realize halfway through that some part of it is missing. Never again will you be driving your hospital projects by the seat of your pants, hoping everything will come together.

"In business, knowing is a manager and hope is for fools."

CHAPTER 7

THE ULTIMATE BENEFIT

**"Wishers wish, hopers hope;
but the successful manager
just gets it done."**

By now, many of you may be saying to yourself, "I haven't got the time to do the self-evaluation. Yes, it's a good idea, but it just takes too long." I empathize and I understand. You want to do the self-evaluation but can't find the time to do it! Listen very carefully: Do it! Just do it! The factor that always differentiates those who succeed from those who do not is that the successful person just does whatever is necessary to get the job done. That's not to say that there aren't ways to get the job done that will take some of the pressure off. There are. In this chapter, I'm going to share with you ways to get the self-evaluation done without overly stressing about it and without putting everything else in your life on hold while you do it.

Three Ways to Do Your Self-Evaluation

Basically, there are three ways to accomplish the self-evaluation. The first way is the approach I suspect most of you are contemplating —namely, doing it yourself. You are envisioning blocking off three or four days of your time to do it. That is one way. If you have a small practice that doesn't require your constant attention, doing it yourself might be an option. If you opt to do it yourself, there are a couple of factors to keep in mind.

First, the self-evaluation process will take you at least three or four days, maybe more. Second, when you do it by yourself, you get a tunnel-vision view of your practice. That is to say, you only see things through your eyes. Is that so bad? Maybe not. But to get a true picture of your practice, wouldn't it be better to get the views of more than just one set of eyes? As we'll discuss later in this chapter, I believe that the more minds you can involve, the better result you'll achieve. I assume, however, that most of you are an integral part of your practice. You need to be there to help ensure the success of your practice. Taking several days off to do the self-evaluation just won't work! Consequently, this option just is not a viable one for most people.

The second option is similar to the first: You do it yourself, but you do it over a period of time using a planned, systematic approach. It might take you two weeks or two months. The truth is it really doesn't matter how long it takes to complete the self-evaluation. What is important is that you find a way to do it. Build a timetable that will give you the confidence you need to accomplish this huge task. If you take this option, you still have total control over the process, but you spread the work out over a period of time. It's not necessary to do it all at once; the important thing is to get it done. If it takes you a month or more to do it, fine. Once again, though, the primary drawback to this method is that it provides a one-dimensional view of the practice.

Jack Stack, CEO of the Springfield Manufacturing Corporation and author of the book *The Great Game of Business,* noted that it is easy to stop one person, but it is almost impossible to stop a hundred people. That thought is very profound, especially in the veterinary industry, where the owner traditionally has retained total control of the practice and rarely has shared any details with the employees. My interpretation of Jack Stack's statement is that it advocates a management style that is grounded in the owner's or manager's ability to get the employees involved in the business—in other words, to set the stage for getting the employees to "buy in" to the course you set for the practice. Now, I'm not advocating that a hundred people do your self-evaluation. Nor am I advocating that you give up control of your business to your employees. But getting your employees involved will bring about positive results you may not be able to imagine now. This philosophy brings us to the third option.

The third option touches on a topic that I've been talking about throughout the book: achieving the employee buy-in. You accomplish this goal by assigning portions of the self-evaluation to a number of employees who are then responsible for performing portions of the self-evaluation. Just last year when it was time to do the self-evaluation, I gathered my management group together—the hospital director, my office manager, the receptionist team leader, and my two technician team leaders. (We needed two veterinary technician supervisors because we ran a 24-hour, 7-day a week facility with more than 30 veterinary technicians, veterinary technician assistants, and kennel helpers.) Each person on the management team was assigned a portion of the self-evaluation. We then created a timetable for completion. Each week, at our managers meeting, I received updates of their progress. We also discussed the findings and answered questions they had regarding certain aspects of the evaluation.

The Benefit of Dividing the Job

When I did this, several important things happened. The first, and perhaps the most obvious, result was that it took the burden of doing the entire self-evaluation off my shoulders. I was still charged with the responsibility of getting it done, but by delegating portions of the job to my section managers, I was free to do other essential tasks. I lifted the weight of the job off my shoulders when I got the other managers to help. The second, and perhaps most important, result was the feeling I generated in my managers.

You are probably thinking that my employees hated me because I gave them more work to do. The truth is, my managers felt great about the situation! Here I was, a hospital administrator, asking for their help. I was trusting them to do a very important job. I had faith in their abilities. I was openly asking them to give me their views and input about the hospital operations. The impact of delegating portions of the self-evaluation to them was very powerful. They took this responsibility very seriously because I was trusting them to do a very important job. It motivated them and boosted their egos—it was as if I had given them a generous compliment. When I asked for their help, I was telling them that I had faith in them and that I trusted them. It was, indeed, a generous compliment!

There were even more positive consequences. My managers followed suit with their sections. As they were doing their portions of the self-evaluation, they routinely solicited opinions and information from the rest of the staff. The same feelings I was able to give my managers, they cultivated in the rest of the employees. To a lesser degree, the entire staff was involved in the self-evaluation, and all the employees were motivated by the fact that our management group was asking for their input. The entire process took us about a month. When all the parts were put together, it became a living, breathing document that represented the views, opinions, and data of most of the staff members. The staff was very proud of our accomplishments and recognized the weaknesses that many of them had pointed out.

Of course, when you get all the pieces of the evaluation together, you must edit it and adjust it to represent your vision of the practice's future. It is, after all, your business and your big picture that you want the evaluation to represent. Once the evaluation was completed, I shared it with the employees at a general staff meeting. As I was going through it, I could hear people say, "I found that problem." Pride filled the room. The entire staff was uplifted and motivated. They found the problems, and by gosh, they were going to fix them.

As I turned the strategic plan into the tactical plan, volunteers came out of the woodwork to help fix things. I had achieved employee buy-in! Because the staff was involved in the self-evaluation process and had a sense of belonging to the system, they were ready, willing, and able to contribute wholeheartedly to repairing the problems. They no longer felt like pawns being pushed around. Instead, they felt like part of the process, and because they were part of the process, they readily accepted the need to fix it.

A word of caution: Employees are smart. They can see a phony a mile away. When you delegate responsibility, you must do it completely, and you must trust your employees to do a good job. If they don't know how to do it, show them how before you set them loose. If you use this method of completing your self-evaluation, you must not micromanage and look over your employees' shoulders every step of the way. If you do, you will have the opposite effect. Instead of instilling a sense of pride and confidence, you will cultivate distrust and a feeling of antagonism.

Summary

The task of completing the self-evaluation may be more than you want to take on by yourself. There is a great advantage to dividing the job up among your staff. If you've never tried this method of management or have never involved your staff in a large evaluative process, I encourage you to do so. If you are sincere, the benefits you'll reap will astound you. You will see them in both the evolution of the culture in your hospital and, because you have such a motivated staff, in your bottom line!

CHAPTER 8

THE FINAL WORD

"Success is not an accident. If you don't plan for it, it probably won't happen."

In this small book we have covered a lot of material, and it may be difficult to visualize how all of it fits into place. I'll now bring it all together and show you how the process flows from the first step in strategic planning to the last nail on the barn door in tactical plans. Once you've seen the total picture, you'll realize that the time invested in following a formal planning process will pay you back tenfold in confidence, peace of mind, and profits! So, let's take it from the top!

Recapitulation

To understand the total planning process, one must accept the fact that planning is a fundamental management principle. You must believe that you can't properly manage any business without a basic knowledge of planning. With that knowledge comes the inherent responsibility to the business: a responsibility to perform better, produce more efficiently, and, of course, to increase profitability. In your quest to be more efficient and profitable, you begin by writing your strategic plan.

The strategic plan begins with a detailed self-evaluation, which you do for a number of reasons. First and foremost, your self-evaluation—a vision quest—will help you set your goals for the practice as well as define the level of achievement you aspire to. A self-evaluation also gives you baseline data needed to forecast the future and the opportunity to regain control over your practice. You probably decided to read this book because you were tired of running around and putting out fires every day, tired of those important jobs being forgotten or put on the back burner because there was just not enough time to do them. When you are distracted and tasks do not get done, you lose productive time and, consequently, profits. Self-evaluations, you remember, must be done with an open mind and an honest heart. Anything less is just an exercise in futility. When you complete your self-evaluation, strengths and weaknesses are identified. With this information in hand, you write your assessment. Now you have a firm understanding of what's happening in your practice; others can read your self-evaluation and know what's going on.

Once you've completed your self-evaluation, it's time to move on to the next step in strategic planning: creating an action list. Your action list, which focuses on the execution of your goals, is a compilation of every project you want to do. You take your weaknesses, assign an action verb to them, and plug the item into the list. You also ascertain your goals on the basis of the baseline data, which you derived from the self-evaluation; thus, you can forecast your goals for the coming year. It's important to remember, first, that action list items must be active; use an action verb to describe what you are going to do. Second, set realistic start dates and completion dates. It does no good if you set unrealistic start or completion dates. Last, you will assign people to accomplish the jobs. Assign one person the primary responsibility for completing a project and another (secondary) person who can be the back-up for the project or can help get the job done. Remember that an action list is not written in any particular order. Items can be put in the template as they come off the self-evaluation. An action list does, however, begin the process of prioritizing your work and is also the key tool for making the transition into tactical plans. And through your tactical plans, the day-to-day work gets accomplished.

❝*If you want to see the world,
ask for a strategic plan, but if
you only want to see a single
country, ask for a tactical plan.***❞**

As you make the transition from the strategic plan to your tactical plans, you must understand the difference between them. The strategic plan paints the big picture of the practice; the tactical plans break down the picture into bite-sized pieces. Tactical plans make it easier for us to handle the myriad jobs we must deal with every day.

The transition from strategic plans to tactical plans is simple. In essence, you did it when you wrote your action list. The action list becomes a tactical plan when you reorganize it and put it into a time frame. Remember, a tactical plan is based on time. There are two types of tactical plans: quarterly master action plans (QMAPs) and monthly tactical action plans (MTAPs). The key word *action*, which describes both of these plans, is the fundamental principle of tactical plans. As we begin the transition from strategic plans to tactical plans, we use the QMAPs—action lists put into a time frame based on calendar quarters. QMAPs not only formalize your priorities, but they also provide a basis for putting your action list into a format that you can use to accomplish your tasks. In addition, QMAPs, which break your goals and projects down one step further, are used to develop your MTAPs.

There are two types of MTAPs: grocery lists and comprehensive plans. Both take your goals and projects to the working level; MTAPs are a powerful tool that give you the power to control what you do in any given day. Consequently, you are bound to be more productive and more profitable.

Grocery lists give a manager the flexibility to select what will happen daily, weekly, or monthly. If you simply write down what you want to do during a period of time, your grocery list will keep you on track for starting projects and will keep you from forgetting the dreary day-to-day activities we all face.

Comprehensive tactical plans will keep you from having a coronary! Of all the plans there are, comprehensive plans are perhaps the least used, which is strange because they are the most compelling reason for planning. If you have a comprehensive plan, all the guesswork about a project or goal disappears and there are only answers. Unhappily, many managers at all levels either don't know how to use a comprehensive plan or are too lazy to do so. A comprehensive plan breaks a multifaceted project down into its individual components and defines it. We are frequently faced with projects that pose many questions: Who is going to do it? How much will it cost? What type of advertising will we do? How will we track the project's success? The important thing to remember about comprehensive plans is that they tell us everything we need to know about a project, when and how to accomplish it, and how much it will cost.

So as you move from the strategic plan to the tactical plan, the process remains the same. You take the big picture and begin to break it down until you have pieces that are big enough to swallow. In other words, you make the job easy to manage. That's what planning is all about. Making a mountain into a molehill. Transforming the big picture into a manageable, workable size. If you want to accomplish your goals, you must plan to do so.

> **❝We all know two brains are better than one, but a half-dozen brains are unstoppable!❞**

If your employees are encouraged to take an active role in evaluating the practice, they will feel that they are part of the process and that they can be part of the solution. One of the keys for achieving this desirable situation is the "buy in." Be sure your employees believe what you're saying and what you're trying to do.

> **❝If you plan to be a great manager, you better learn to manage a great plan!❞**

Conclusion

Planning is one of the primary functions of management. It is incumbent upon us, as managers, to constantly refine and improve our management skills. By necessity, this includes our ability to plan effectively. Over the years, veterinary professionals have made great strides in improving systems for both delivery of care to companion animals and managing a practice.

Management is a never-ending journey of learning and adjusting. Properly equipping ourselves with the right tools for the job means learning everything we can about planning. The more you know, the more you practice planning, the sooner your practice will show higher efficiencies that will lead naturally to higher profits. Therefore, I leave you with a final thought: If you can work in a field you love and make a decent profit, isn't it worth the extra effort? My answer is a resounding Yes.

> **❝ I didn't hope I would be successful. I planned it!❞**

APPENDIX A

SELF-EVALUATION CHECKLIST

Significant accomplishments _____

Market environment _____

Competition _____

1.0 Hospital Structure, Leadership, and Management

- •Organizational chart drawn _____

- •Organizational chart used _____

- •Organizational structure assessed _____

1.1 Job descriptions in place for each position _____

- •Skill levels and job tasks defined for each position _____

- •Roles and responsibilities defined and clear to employees _____
_____

- •Are employees clear on what outcomes they are to create for the hospital?
_____

- •Do employees have clear "line of sight" of how they fit into the big picture?
_____

- •Are performance objectives defined and clear to employees? _____
_____

1.2 Leadership and management assessment of the effectiveness of each member of the management team

- •Hospital director _____

- •Manager _____

- •Team leaders _____

1.3 Planning assessment

- •Strategic business plan and annual budget in place _____

- •Quarterly tactical plan and project list review_____

- •Monthly plan and project list review _____

1.4 Implementation

- •Use of defined objective list and action plan project list_____

- •Is there a basis for action? _____

- •Does the management team work on the business as well as in the business? _____

- •Are the prioritized projects completed on time? _____

1.5 Performance measurement and evaluation

- •Monthly financial reports analyses by management team _____
_____

•Action plan project list review _____

•Ensure the use of an action plan project list that includes project description, short action plan outline, person responsible, budget impact, and date of completion _____

•Review progress of projects since last management meeting _____
_____

•Evaluate process for adding and prioritizing new projects _____

•Evaluate process for defining new problems or issues that need immediate attention _____
_____

•Problem-solve for best solutions with the management team _____
_____

•Create action plan with date of completion and person responsible and add to project list _____

•Reprioritize the list with the new additions after each management team meeting _____

•Evaluate feedback and accountability _____
_____

•Are there weekly hospital team meetings? _____

•Are the meetings efficient (no longer than 1–1.5 hours with defined agenda)? _____

•How is the feedback communicated? _____

_____

•Do team members feel responsible for hospital performance? _____

_____

•How are they held accountable? _____

_____

1.6 Team-hospital culture

•Assess commitment to mission _____

_____

•Assess hospital team for ability to perform the technical skills and the interpersonal skills of their jobs _____

_____

•Evaluate training and education _____

•Assess compensation _____

•Is the compensation process competitive for the market area?

_____

•Is there a bonus system? _____

•Assess recruiting and hiring _____

•Employee turnover _____

•Employee turnover as percentage of total employees _____

•Assess employee morale _____

•Assess ability of doctors, technicians, CSRs, and others to develop effective client and team relationships:

   •Doctors _____

   •Technicians _____

   •CSRs _____

   •Others _____

1.7 Assess training and education of new employees

   •Indoctrination of new employees into the hospital culture_____
   _____

   •Does the employee have and understand the employee manual? ____
   _____

1.8 Assess training and education in the following areas:

   •Leadership and management training _____

   •Functional, technical, and production training for each position ____
   _____

   •Cross-training process especially between the technicians and the CSRs _____

•Client service training_____

2.0 Client Service Delivery System

2.1 Development of long-term client relationships

•Client retention rate _____

•Active client base _____

•New client numbers_____

•Average wait time for appointment _____

•Client satisfaction score/client services surveys _____

•Empathy for both the pet and the client _____

•Responsiveness to both the pet's and client's needs_____

•Reliability of our implied promises to the client _____
_____

•Do we demonstrate assurance through our competence creating "quality in perception" in the client's mind? _____

•Assess intangibles (such as the image of our people and facility) ____
_____

2.2 Hospital admission process assessment

• Estimates given for all cases _____

• Accounts receivable (AR) arrangements made before work performed

_____

• Drop-off service availability _____

• Appointment process and ability to handle walk-in clients _____

_____

• Timeliness of doctor to appointment time _____

• Assessment of admission process relative to wait time _____

_____

2.3 Hospital release process assessment

• Bill matches estimate _____

• Chart, medications, and pet prepared and ready for client arrival ____

_____

• Clean pet on release _____

• Discharge appointment with doctor for every hospitalized case _____

_____

• Discharge instructions for each case _____

• Follow-up plan _____

•Recall process _____

•Hospital initiates follow-up phone call on each medical and surgical case _____

•Recheck appointments made for medical and surgical cases that warrant a follow-up exam _____

•Reminders for medical follow-up as necessary _____

•Assessment of discharge process relative to wait time _____
_____

•In-hospital patient status update _____

•Lab or other diagnostic results updated as necessary _____

3.0 Phone Call and Message Management

•Assess telephone management_____

•Assess phone skills _____

•Assess management of hold time. Is there music or a message on hold?
_____

•Are phone calls returned in a timely manner?_____

•Is the appointment scheduling process efficient? _____

•Are clients able to make an appointment within 24 hours or sooner?
_____

4.0 Communication of Information About Pet from Work Center

- To CSRs and between the technicians and doctors as well as between shifts _____

- Hospital announcements to the staff—memos and bulletin board ____
  _____

- Client management process—building long-term relationships _____
  _____

- Client referral program _____

- Client recovery process—specific scenario training to deal with an unhappy client _____

- Emotional support for client upon the loss of pet _____

- Wait time management process—queuing theory in place to reduce the perception of the wait time _____

- Sound and noise control _____

- Is there a client education process (handouts, seminars, etc.)? _____
  _____

- Is there a specific children's education program?_____

- Is there a special area for children in the reception area? _____
  _____

- Are school tours conducted? _____

5.0 Image Assessment

5.1 Friendly and professional image of:

• Sign _____

• Grounds and parking lot _____

• Facility _____

• Exterior _____

• Interior _____

• Staff _____

• Printed materials _____

5.2 Assessment of cleanliness of:

• Grounds and parking lot _____

• Facility _____

• Exterior _____

• Interior _____

• Staff _____

• Pets _____

5.3 Quality care and quality control

• Procedure ratios assessment—ratios of various procedures per exam room visits _____

• Chart review by medical director_____

• Assess client compliance to doctor recommendation _____

• Doctor average client charge (ACC)_____

• Assessment of quality care and quality control _____

• Assess exam room technique of doctors and technicians _____

_____

• Assess rounds and doctor communication with each other on case (case hand-offs)_____

• Use of specialists when necessary _____

• Assess training and continuing education _____

• Standard medical library in place and used_____

• Hospital supplied with minimum standard medical equipment and instruments necessary to produce competent care _____

_____

5.4 Growth-production system

- Assess production system _____

- Assess production by doctor _____

- Assess pricing _____

- Assess fee capture_____

- Assess hospital facility _____

5.5 Hospital performance

- Revenue or hospital production _____

- Revenue growth compared to previous year _____

- Number of transactions _____

- Transaction growth compared to previous year _____

- Average transaction charge (ATC) for hospital_____

- ATC for hospital compared to previous year _____

- Doctor production _____

- Doctor average client charge (ACC)_____

- Number of new clients _____

•Number of new clients compared to previous year_____

•Recheck ratio (ratio of number of rechecks to number of exams) _____

_____

•Utilization rate (hospital visits per patient per year) _____

•Reminder compliance (percentage of patient base current on vaccinations) _____

5.6 Services offered

•Medical and surgical services _____

•Well-care services at market pricing _____

•Annual physical exam program _____

•Vaccination clinics _____

•Spay and neuter clinics _____

•Dental clinics _____

•Primary care assessment (services common to most practices) _____

_____

•Sophisticated care and use of specialist assessment_____

•Emergency care service assessment _____

- Ancillary services _____

    - Boarding _____

    - Grooming and bathing _____

    - Adoption program _____

    - Obedience training _____

- Assess hospital convenience_____

    - Days of operation _____

    - Hours of operation _____

6.0 Key Marketing Functions

- Reminder for annual physical exam and vaccinations_____

- Recall program on all surgical and medical cases _____

- Recheck program on all appropriate cases _____

- Hospital brochure _____

- Hospital newsletter _____

- Phone shopper capture process _____

- Client referral process _____

• New client program in place _____

• New client follow-up letter from hospital _____

• Brochure to each new client _____

• Other appropriate hospital information, tour, etc., to each new client
_____

• Yellow page advertising _____

• Well-care program _____

• Pet shop program _____

• Humane work program _____

• Community work/relationships _____

• Marketing calendar in use _____

• Client education process _____

• Client and children education program _____

• Condolence letter signed by staff for each client that has lost a pet __
_____

7.0 Production System Assessment

• Production by doctor _____

- Are doctors trained and do they use the steps to a successful exam room visit? _____

- Do doctors provide answers for the client's problem? _____

- Revenue production by doctor _____

- Average charge per client by doctor_____

- Number of clients seen by doctor _____

- Evaluation of fee sensitivity by doctor_____

- Pricing review _____

- Pricing of key services _____

- Itemization process _____

- Fee capture and assessment_____

- Chart pricing process _____

- Use of estimates _____

- Discharge preparation of in-hospital patient chart _____

- Hospital facility assessment _____

•Facility capacity for producing high-quality veterinary medical services_____

•Facility capacity for producing high-quality ancillary services _____
_____

8.0 Financial Assessment

•Operating cash flow (OCF) _____

•OCF before rent _____

•Direct costs _____

•Total labor _____

•Total labor per hospital transaction _____

•Total indirect costs (excluding rent) _____

•Rent _____

•Accounts receivable _____

•Deposits-to-sales ratio _____

9.0 Management Issues Assessment

•Work center productivity_____

•Review scheduling of paraprofessionals process _____

- Review scheduling of doctors process _____

- Assess efficiency of work center _____

- Use of treatment board to track work _____

9.1 Inventory system assessment

- Ordering and price comparison process (once a week) _____

- Inventory on hand (about 1 week's supply for most products) _____
  _____

9.2 Production and productivity control

- Weekly labor hour assessment as compared to scheduled hours
  budget _____

- Overtime assessment _____

- Budget control sheets for direct expenses _____

- Evaluation of work-flow efficiency and capacity of the hospital
  facility _____

10.0 Baseline Statistics Summary

- Operating cash flow (OCF) (as percentage of net revenue) _____
  _____

•OCF before rent (as percentage of net revenue) _____

•Direct costs (as percentage of net revenue) _____

•Drugs and supplies (as percentage of medical services) _____
_____

•Laboratory costs _____

  •Inside laboratory _____

  •Outside laboratory _____

•Premium food cost _____

•Retail cost_____

•Total labor (as percentage of net hospital revenue) _____

•Total labor per hospital transaction _____

•Doctor and veterinary technician compensation per medical service transaction _____

•Doctor and veterinary technician compensation as percentage of medical revenue _____

•Support labor per hospital transaction _____

•Support labor as percentage of net hospital revenue _____

- Total indirect costs (excluding rent) _____

- Maintenance and repair expenses _____

- Office supply expenses_____

- Other expenses _____

- Rent _____

- New equipment _____

- Medical production per doctor _____

- Transactions per doctor _____

- Accounts receivable _____
  _____

- Bad debt and write-off loss (percentage against total revenue) _____
  _____

- Deposits-to-sales ratio (deposits as percentage of sales) _____
  _____

Appendix B

TOP 300 Things to Do

Marketing

first reminders

second reminders

third reminders

yellow page advertisements

referral reports

referral letters

customer newsletters

send new clients letters/coupons

send sympathy cards

referral veterinarian newsletter

target marketing

mining old records

changing the front sign

tracking coupons

checking new schemes

tracking phone shopper successes

Payroll

time-card computations

fix entries/mistakes

doctor salary commutations

record doctor numbers in computer

update figures in budget

maintain payroll binder/reports

Mail

> refill meter
>
> track meter
>
> equipment maintenance
>
> incoming distribution
>
> outgoing postage/evaluate for theft

New Personnel Processing

> complete INS form 9
>
> complete W-4 form
>
> review benefits package
>
> complete benefit forms
>
> establish computer time card
>
> establish cashier code
>
> establish training record
>
> establish personnel file

Office Functions

> maintain masters of all forms
>
> monitor usage of forms in hospital/Lodge/grooming
>
> establish order quantity
>
> place orders/pick up
>
> order business cards
>
> track office supply usage
>
> develop/use office supply purchase order
>
> evaluate purchases/prices
>
> maintain office copier/supplies
>
> coordinate repair/maintenance
>
> maintain printers and supplies
>
> file medical records
>
> call appointments the day before

pull/set-up file for next day's appointments

verify phone/address

print daily appointment list every few hours

purge files at_____years

call clients prior to purging

change light bulbs inside

change light bulbs outside

change light bulbs in sign

update employee phone numbers

maintain phone code log

Reports

daily

    run day sheet

    run daily check register

    run daily credit card report

    balance cash/checks/credit cards with reports

    do deposit slip

    get deposit to bank

    maintain report book

monthly

    run monthly reports

    make copy of monthly reports

    put reports in binder

yearly

    run yearly reports

    make copy of yearly reports

    put report in binder

Computer Operations

      ensure daily/monthly/yearly backup

      store tapes properly

      add/change employee information

      add/change clinic information

      maintain network connections

      maintain terminal integrity

      adjust/maintain print queue

      interact with software support

      interact with hardware support

Building Maintenance

      call air conditioner repair

      call electric repair

      call roof repair

      call insurance for claims

      get bids for projects/repairs

      call plumber for repairs

      call medical equipment repair

      call anesthesia repair/maintenance

      call X-ray maintenance/repair

      call processor maintenance/repair

      call for sign repair

      evaluate lawn maintenance

      inspect building/grounds for damage

      inspect outside for cleanliness

      inspect windows for damage

      ensure doors/locks function properly

      evaluate floor cleaning contract work

      evaluate housekeeping work

Medical Systems

       nosicomial infection control measures

       medical waste control

       waste anesthetic gas control

       hazardous chemical disposal

       sharps disposal

       body disposal

       order oxygen

       liquid oxygen tank controls

       bottle oxygen controls

       ethylene oxide controls

       autoclave maintenance

       sterilization procedures

       put together sterile packs

       maintain pack lists

       cold pack lists

       maintain endoscope

       maintain ultrasound

       maintain intensive care unit

       maintain air compressor

       maintain dental unit

       maintain ozone emitters

       maintain treatment room cabinets

       maintain laboratory cabinets

       maintain examination room cabinets

       maintain examination room refrigerators

       maintain client handouts

       stock scrub room

       fill isoflorane vaporizers

       maintain clipper/blades

       maintain/calibrate laboratory equipment

run periodic quality control tests

coordinate periodic X-ray quality control

maintain X-ray log

review film badge reports

maintain surgery log

do laundry (hospital)

do laundry (groom/Lodge)

keep retail stocked

stock pet food

stock treatment area

stock ultrasound room

maintain X-ray films/files

maintain computerized tomography/magnetic resonance image files

maintain endoscope videos

clean waiting area/kids area

clean receptionist area

clean front office

clean/maintain front stock room

clean front restrooms

clean parking lot

clean around bushes

clean examination rooms

clean laboratory area

clean pharmacy area

clean treatment room

clean ward A

clean ward B

clean ward C

clean ward D

clean holding room

clean X-ray/processing room

clean ultrasound room

clean surgery room 1

clean surgery room 2

clean scrub room

clean preparation/autoclave room

clean administration office

clean break room

clean conference room

clean business office

clean bath/grooming rooms

clean Lodge reception

clean Lodge

Inventory Management

check-in products (drugs and supplies)

verify invoice

update prices in computer

enter cost in checkbook

enter costs in scorecard

invoice disposition

update stock/order levels

generate computer purchase orders

verify inventory with computer totals

monitor/inventory controlled drugs

order control drug forms

update/review control drug log

monitor in-house use of drugs/supplies

check in products (pet food)

verify invoices

update prices

enter costs in checkbook

      enter cost in scorecard

      invoice disposition

      generate computer order

      track in-house use (hospital)

      track in-house use (Lodge)

Management Functions

      schedule periodic training

      schedule section training

      schedule OSHA training

      schedule finance/open book training

      schedule customer service training

      schedule continuing education for everyone

      track training/continuing education by person

      track vacation/sick days

      monitor personnel/training records

      maintain separate Immigration Naturalization Service (INS) file

      review/update treatment protocols

      maintain protocol binder

      review/update standard operating procedures (SOPs)

Recommended Readings

Blanchard, Ken, John P. Carlos, and Alan Randolph. *Empowerment Takes More Than a Minute*. San Francisco: Berrett-Koehler Publishers, 1996.

Boylan, Bob. *Getting Everyone in Your Boat Rowing in the Same Direction*. Holbrook, Mass.: Adams Media Corporation, 1995.

Clark, Ross, DVM. *Mastering the Marketplace: Taking Your Practice to the Top*. Lenexa, Kan.: Veterinary Medicine Publishing Group, 1996.

Stack, Jack. *The Great Game of Business*. New York: Currency/Doubleday Publications, 1992.

ABOUT THE AUTHOR

Born in Chicago and raised in the suburbs of Los Angeles, Brian Hayden joined the U.S. Air Force in 1972, where he was crossed-trained into the veterinary service in 1974. From 1977 to 1982, Hayden was stationed at Hessich Oldendorf Air Station in Germany. In this post, Hayden served as the sole veterinary technician, establishing and operating a veterinary public health laboratory. In 1982, Hayden was assigned to Brooks Air Force Base in San Antonio where he was a master instructor in the Environmental Health Branch of U.S. Air Force School of Aerospace Medicine. In 1987, the Air Force posted Hayden to England where he served as superintendent of Aerospace Medicine Service, a branch of the force's medical facility located at (Royal Air Force) Greenham Common. In this position, he worked closely with the hospital administrator.

A heart attack in 1989 abruptly ended Hayden's military career. However, with his background as a veterinary technician and his experience managing medical facilities, he was soon running two small veterinary clinics outside San Antonio. In 1993, he moved to southern California to be the administrator of a 24-hour veterinary facility. By 1994, Hayden was managing and consulting for a partnership that owned four hospitals in California.

In January 1997, National PetCare Centers hired Hayden to be the administrator of its largest hospital—a 16,500 sq. ft, 24-hour facility, which provides general practice services, a specialty referral practice, and an emergency practice, with boarding and grooming. As administrator, Hayden's responsibilities included developing strategic and tactical plans and budgets, forecasting production and financial data, performing statistical analysis and evaluation of production systems, and ensuring effective implementation of hospital and corporate policies.

In March 1999, Hayden established Hayden Management Group (HMG), a veterinary practice consulting service headquartered in Euless, Texas.

Hayden has served on AAHA's Management Associate Committee. Married for 25 years, he has two grown children and one grandson.